Sugar Detox
IN 10 DAYS

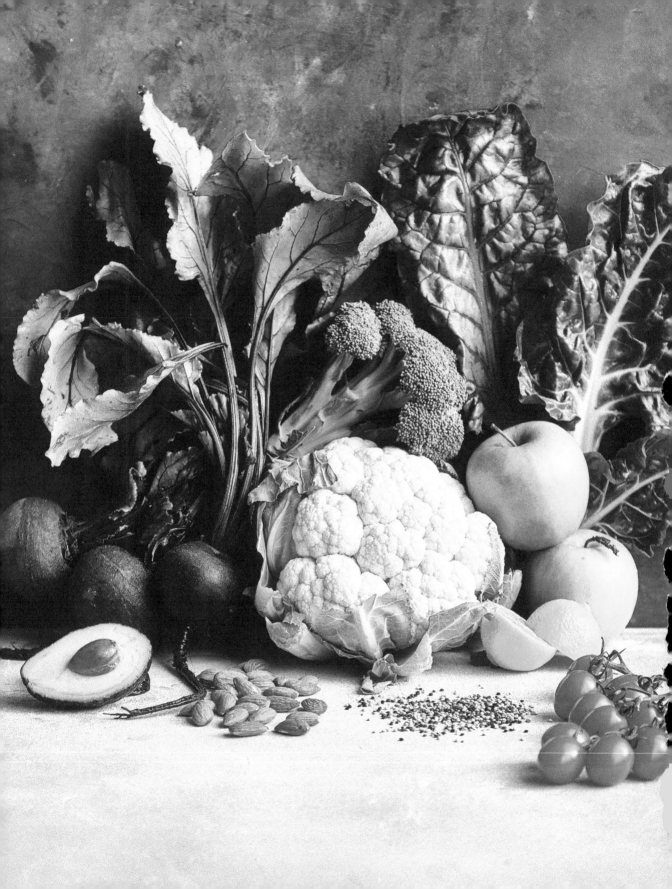

Sugar Detox
IN 10 DAYS

100+ RECIPES TO HELP
ELIMINATE SUGAR CRAVINGS

Pam Rocca

PHOTOGRAPHY BY HÉLÈNE DUJARDIN

ROCKRIDGE
PRESS

For general information on our other products and services or to obtain technical support, please contact our Customer Care Department within the United States at (866) 744-2665, or outside the United States at (510) 253-0500.

Rockridge Press publishes its books in a variety of electronic and print formats. Some content that appears in print may not be available in electronic books, and vice versa.

Interior and Cover Designer: Lisa Schreiber

Art Producer: Sara Feinstein

Editor: Daniel Grogan

Production Manager: Jose Olivera

Production Editor: Melissa Edeburn

Photography © 2020 Hélène Dujardin; Evi Abeler, p. ix.

Food styling by Anna Hampton.

Author photo courtesy of © Nat Caron.

ISBN: Print 978-1-64611-752-9 | eBook 978-1-64611-753-6

R0

This book is dedicated to you, the reader, and every person who is committed to improving their health and investing in their happiness.

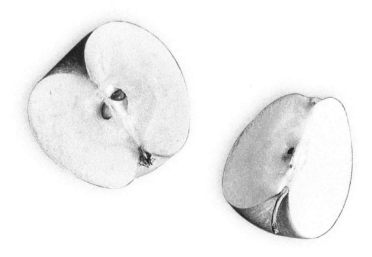

Contents

Introduction

Welcome to your sugar detox meal plan. I am so excited to help you transform the way you eat in as little as 10 days!

This book will teach you tips and tricks to help you kick your sugar addiction and cravings to the curb. It will show you where sugar lurks, why and how to eliminate it from your diet, and how to give your pantry a sugar-decreasing makeover. It presents four meal plans as well as shopping lists so you can tailor your sugar detox to your nutritional preferences and goals.

The detox may seem daunting, but the results will make the effort well worth it. By removing sugar and refined foods from your diet, you can experience an increase in your energy level and alertness and a reduction in bloating and inflammation. Other benefits include weight loss, improved complexion, and better sleep, digestion, and blood sugar balance. You may even fall in love with cooking again.

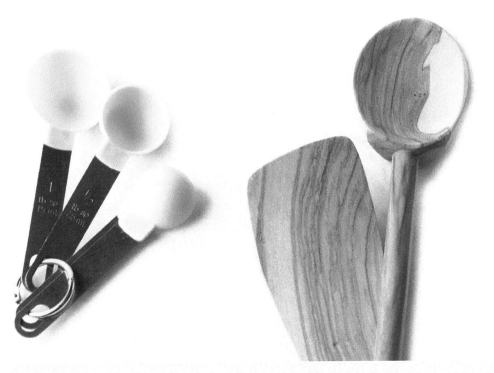

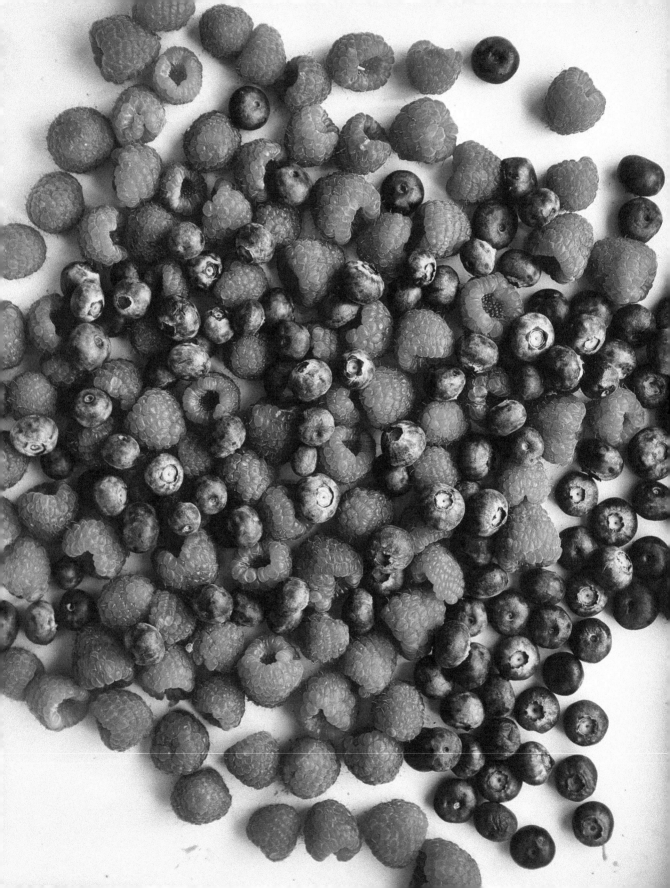

1

The Unsweetened Truth About Sugar

Sugar is hidden in many foods and beverages, and it can be hard to recognize just how much we are consuming on a daily basis. Sugar is also addictive and can lead to health conditions like obesity and type 2 diabetes. This chapter describes the effects of sugar and how to recognize if you are a sugar addict. You will also find out how stress can hinder your healthy eating goals and will learn to uncover healthy ways to manage stress without reaching for food.

Sugar Cravings and Effects

When you consume sugar, your body releases the "feel good" neurotransmitter dopamine. Dopamine promotes feelings of reward and pleasure, so the more sugar you consume, the better you feel. The problem is that the "good" feeling is temporary, and it will inevitably leave you craving more dopamine and more sugar. This craving would not be detrimental if you were getting naturally occurring sugar from nutrient-dense whole-food sources like strawberries and mangos. The problem is that today foods containing refined sugar are all around us, and most are "nutrient dead." The first step in kicking a sugar habit is learning what sugar is and how it affects your body.

When you think of sugar, you're likely thinking of the white, granular kind often used in baking, but this is only one type of sugar. Depending on its chemical structure, sugar can be classified as one of three forms:

1. Monosaccharides (one sugar molecule): glucose, dextrose, fructose—also known as a simple sugar or simple carbohydrate

2. Disaccharides (two sugar molecules = two monosaccharides combined): sucrose, maltose, lactose

3. Polysaccharides (many monosaccharides bonded together): complex sugars or complex carbohydrates, such as starch

Each form of sugar functions differently in the body. Simple carbohydrates get broken down in the body and into the bloodstream quickly. They are great if you need energy immediately, but they can also cause a spike in blood sugar, followed by a fast crash, which can soon lead you to want more sugar or food. By contrast, complex carbohydrates (such as beans and gluten-free whole grains) take longer to break down and digest, providing energy throughout the day. So if you want to lose weight, it's important to consume more healthy complex carbohydrates, especially ones that come from vegetables and contain fiber.

Perils of Refined Sugars

Refined sugar contains calories (energy) but doesn't provide vitamins, minerals, antioxidants, or healthy proteins. When we consume too much sugar, the liver converts the excess into glycogen; when the glycogen builds up, it gets converted into fat. This fat accumulates in our hips, belly, thighs, and elsewhere and can lead to serious health conditions. But sugar does more than just make us gain weight. Some short-term effects of excessive sugar consumption are fatigue, mood swings, muscle fatigue, acne, food addictions, inflammation, disrupted sleep, premenstrual symptoms, and painful periods. Some long-term effects are depression, anxiety, insomnia, insulin resistance or type 2 diabetes, obesity or weight gain, inflammation, and adrenal fatigue.

Where Sugar Lurks

Sugar is hidden in so many of our foods and beverages you may not even realize just how much you are consuming every day. Begin to read food labels and ingredients lists to see how much sugar is in the foods that you eat regularly. Sugar can be lurking in foods that you may have thought were healthy up to this point. Check out "Different Names for Sugar" (see page 5) to see various ways sugar may be listed on food labels.

WHITE FLOUR

White flour is another refined food. There are three parts to whole grain: the bran (fiber), germ (nutrient dense), and endosperm. When refined white flour is made, the healthy bran and germ are removed, leaving only the starchy endosperm. By removing the nutrient-dense bran and germ, you are left with a food that has little to no nutritional value. Just like refined sugars, refined grains are simple carbohydrate foods that get broken down quickly and easily. This creates a rapid spike in your blood sugar levels, making you feel hungrier sooner, which can lead to eating more calories than your body actually needs. The health effects of consuming white flour on a regular basis may include weight gain, blood sugar imbalances, type 2 diabetes, inflammation, and digestive problems.

DAIRY

This detox eliminates dairy for several reasons. First, all milk has naturally occurring sugars called lactose. Second, many milk and dairy products contain not only lactose, but also added sugar, which is not ideal for a sugar detox. Third, dairy products contain casein and whey protein, which are common allergens. Fourth, some dairy can cause inflammation in the body, which can trigger blood sugar imbalances.

"HEALTHY" FOODS

When you think about sugar in foods, you probably think of sweet treats and desserts, but sugar lurks in a lot of foods considered "healthy." Check out the list below to learn where sugar might be sneaking into your diet.

BOTTLED SMOOTHIES, JUICES, AND KOMBUCHA: These healthy drinks contain a lot of natural and added sugars.

BREAKFAST CEREALS: Yes, even the "healthy" ones like Raisin Bran can have hidden sugar, and when you add milk, the sugar content increases.

GRANOLA BARS AND ENERGY BARS: These bars are often marketed as a healthy snack option but usually contain a ton of sugar.

MUFFINS: Store-bought muffins are typically made with a lot of sugar; check out the recipe for Pumpkin-Spiced Muffins (page 67) to find a homemade, low-sugar replacement.

OATMEAL: Packaged oatmeal can contain a lot of hidden sugars, but don't worry—we offer a healthier, low-sugar option. See the recipe for Baked Oatmeal on page 56.

PASTA SAUCES: Some pasta sauces have a lot of added sugar. You can easily make a healthier option by buying cans of crushed or diced tomatoes.

SALAD DRESSING AND DIPS: Steer clear of creamy dressing. Try making your own low-sugar dressing from one of the recipes in this book (see pages 74 to 78).

YOGURT: Even Greek yogurt can pack a big punch in the sugar department. Think of yogurt, especially flavored options, as ice cream—a sugary treat.

DIFFERENT NAMES FOR SUGAR

When reading nutrition labels, watch out for these ingredients, which are all forms of sugar.

- agave nectar/syrup
- barley malt
- beet sugar
- brown rice syrup
- brown sugar
- cane sugar
- carob sugar
- coconut sugar
- corn sweeteners
- corn syrup
- date sugar/syrup
- dextrose
- evaporated cane juice
- fructose or high-fructose corn syrup
- fruit juice, fruit juice sweeteners, or fruit juice concentrate
- glucose
- golden syrup
- honey
- icing sugar
- invert sugar
- lactose
- maltodextrin
- maltose
- mannitol
- maple syrup
- molasses (or blackstrap molasses)
- palm sugar
- polydextrose
- powdered sugar (or confectioners' sugar)
- raw sugar
- sorbitol
- table sugar (sucrose)
- turbinado sugar (brand name: Sugar in the Raw)
- xylitol

Could You Be a Sugar Addict?

Some seek sugar for the taste, others for the energy or rush, and some to soothe, cope, or deal with stress or emotional upset. If you answer yes to any one of the following questions, then the time to start your 10-day sugar detox is now.

1. Do you need more and more sugar to satisfy a sweet craving?

2. Do you find yourself sneaking or hiding sweet treats?

3. Do you go out of your way to get sugar?

4. Do you eat sweet treats or sugary foods even when you are not hungry?

5. Do you always crave sweets? Have an insatiable sweet tooth?

6. Do you use sugar and sweet foods to cope with difficulties?

7. Do you use sugar to reward yourself?

8. Do you crave comfort foods like breads, pasta, or carb-heavy meals?

9. Do you feel that it's impossible to stop eating your favorite sugary treats?

Stopping Sugar Cravings

The more sugar you take in, the more your body craves it, so when you eliminate it from your system you may experience some withdrawal symptoms. They include headaches, mood swings (as you are no longer getting that dopamine or pleasure burst, you might feel depressed or anxious), restlessness, and changes in sleep patterns. An increase in cravings for carbohydrate-rich foods is also possible.

This book's meal plans will help you mitigate these symptoms while regulating your blood sugar and potentially kickstarting healthy weight loss. Whether you choose the Lean Meat, Pescatarian, Vegan, or Vegetarian plan, you will never feel deprived of satisfying food. The focus is never on what you cannot have, but instead on all the tasty foods you can have.

The Stress–Sugar Connection

Stress is one of the root causes of emotional eating and sugar addictions. When you are stressed, the nervous system sends a message to the adrenal glands to release a hormone called epinephrine, your "fight or flight" hormone. Problems occur when your body is constantly in a stressful state and, as a result, the nervous system releases a hormone called cortisol. Cortisol can increase your appetite, leading to overeating and weight gain. What is even more alarming is that high cortisol and high insulin levels increase cravings for high-fat and sugary foods. Can you see how stress and stress eating can be a vicious cycle?

The following five strategies can help you chill out and find a happy calm.

KEEP A DAILY JOURNAL

To make this 10-day sugar detox even more successful, purchase a journal so you can write down what you are eating and when. Tracking what you are eating will allow you to pick up on any unhealthy patterns or habits. The following are some additional journaling exercises that will help you accomplish your goals in your detox journey.

SHIFT YOUR MINDSET. Write down five "I am" statements or mantras that will help you get in the right mindset to complete this detox. For example, "I am excited to make this healthy new lifestyle change."

FIND YOUR WHY. Journal about your "why." Why do you want to do this detox, and what will happen if you don't make this change in your diet and lifestyle? Why is this detox important to you?

CELEBRATE YOUR WINS AND LEARN FROM FAILURES. The more you focus on how good you feel with your new eating habits, the easier it will be to turn this detox into a healthy lifestyle. If you have a slipup, write about how that feels, why it happened, and how you can plan to do better next time.

CREATE A LIST OF HEALTHY COPING MECHANISMS. You can turn to this list when you find yourself stressed and craving sugar or unhealthy, processed food. Focus on activities that make you feel joyful, relaxed, and satisfied.

MEDITATE

Meditation is scientifically proven to lower both stress and cortisol levels. The best thing is that it can be done anywhere and anytime. There are no rules for how to do it best; you can simply set aside five minutes or more a day and focus on breathing and keeping your mind clear, or you can download a guided meditation that you enjoy. You can practice meditating every morning as part of your routine to start your day in the calmest way possible or do it right before bed to create a healthy nighttime routine and improve your sleep. The idea is to use this tool when you find yourself feeling stressed.

EXERCISE

Exercise is also proven to lower cortisol and stress levels and is very beneficial in several ways when detoxing from sugar. Create a list of physical activities you enjoy and find a way to schedule one or more into your week as a nonnegotiable meeting with yourself to invest in your health. Yoga is an amazing exercise to lower stress levels. If you're not a fan of yoga, try working out with weights, walking outdoors, or biking.

ESTABLISH A ROUTINE

Now that you have created a list of activities you want to do, it's time to set your week up for success. The best way to create impact is to be consistent. What will work best for your schedule so that you can be consistent with your workouts? It does not matter what time of day you work out; the idea is to create a routine that works for you and that you can stick with.

It's important to wait one to two hours after eating to exercise, so plan your workouts around your meals. If you prefer to work out in the morning, try not to eat until after your workout. If you prefer working out in the evening, aim to work out before dinner. If you find yourself hungry, have a light snack 30 to 60 minutes before you exercise.

FIND A BUDDY

This sugar detox is even more successful when it is done with a friend, coworker, or family member. It is an easier and more enjoyable process when the people around you are going through it, too. Having a buddy helps with support and accountability, and you can keep each other on track. You can also cook and meal prep together, work out together, and share healthy strategies for managing stress or sugar cravings.

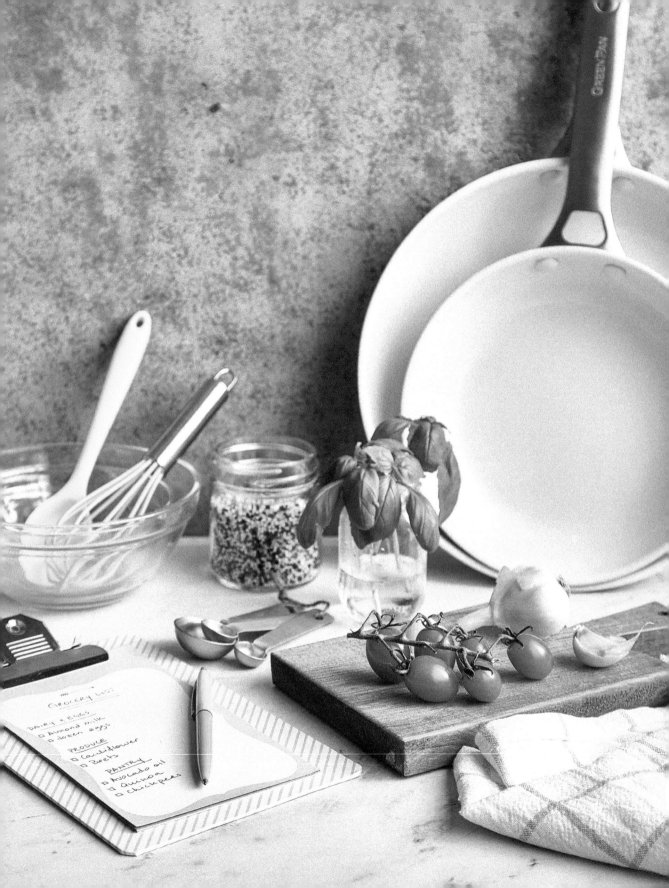

2

Preparing for Your Sugar Detox

Now that you know how harmful sugar can be, let's eliminate it from your diet and kitchen during a 10-day detox. This chapter covers all the wonderful foods that are permitted on this diet, as well as tips on how to make healthy decisions outside of this 10-day detox. If you want to eat healthy, you need to have a healthy kitchen.

Detox for Your Kitchen

There is no better time than right now to give your kitchen and pantry a makeover. By removing all processed, refined, and junk foods, you create space for healthy, nourishing foods that will actually give you energy and make you feel great naturally. Doing a kitchen detox also makes it easier for you to stick to the meal plans in this book.

Begin your makeover with your refrigerator. Empty it and clean every surface. Purge anything past its prime. Remove any processed foods. Shop and restock your refrigerator with foods from your selected meal plan's grocery list.

Next, perk up your pantry. Again, begin by emptying everything and wiping down shelves. Get rid of food that's processed or expired. As you can, invest in different-sized clear jars so foods can easily be organized, viewed, and filled when stock gets low. When you have a well-stocked pantry, you can always whip up a healthy meal and have low-sugar snacks on hand.

Your Sugar Detox Food List

When you nourish your body with nutrient-dense food, you can banish sugar cravings for good. The goal of this detox is to rid the body of toxins that overwhelm your liver, slow down digestion, and contribute to increased blood sugar levels, weight gain, and sluggishness. This plan is loaded with foods and recipes that nourish your body and assist with its natural detoxification process.

COMPLEX WHOLE GRAINS

Unlike other sugar detox books, this book offers meal plans that do not eliminate whole-grain or whole-wheat pasta and unrefined grains. Complex whole grains are complex carbs that contain fiber and that are broken down and digested relatively slowly, which allows your body to maintain healthy blood sugar levels without spikes and crashes. Whole-grain flours are considered "clean" and can be used in moderation throughout the detox. Many other grain-free flours, such as almond flour, chickpea flour, and coconut flour, also can be used.

Complex whole grains include the following:

- Barley
- Brown rice
- Flours (almond, chickpea, and coconut)
- Millet
- Oats
- Quinoa

LEAFY GREENS AND OTHER VEGETABLES

Leafy greens and cruciferous vegetables are detox superstars. They are relatively low in carbohydrates and sugar and are nutrient dense, meaning they contain vitamins, minerals, and phytochemicals. This diet allows some starchy vegetables, but in moderation.

Veggies to include:

- Arugula
- Asparagus
- Bell peppers
- Broccoli
- Brussels sprouts
- Cabbage
- Carrots
- Cauliflower
- Celery
- Collard greens
- Cucumber
- Eggplant
- Garlic
- Ginger
- Kale
- Leeks
- Mixed greens, lettuce, and all leafy greens
- Mushrooms
- Onions
- Parsnips
- Peas
- Spinach
- Squash
- Swiss chard
- Tomatoes
- Zucchini

Starchy vegetables to include in moderation:

- Beets
- Butternut squash
- Spaghetti squash
- Sweet potatoes

HEALTHY FATS

Healthy fats are essential to the body because they help manufacture hormones, protect the heart and other vital organs, improve mood, transport vitamins (A, D, E, and K), and provide insulation. Fats also help keep you full, which is important for weight loss. Contrary to what was once a widely held belief, the right kinds of fats *are* healthy and should be consumed daily.

Foods with healthy fats to include:

- Avocado oil
- Avocados
- Chia seeds
- Coconut oil
- Flax oil
- Flaxseed
- Ghee
- Hemp seeds
- Nuts and seeds
- Extra-virgin olive oil
- Olives
- Salmon
- Toasted sesame oil
- Tuna

LOW-SUGAR FRUITS

Grapefruits and dark berries are high in antioxidants, nutrient dense, and relatively low on the glycemic index, meaning they will not spike your blood sugar or increase your sugar cravings.

Low-sugar fruits to include:

- Bananas (slightly underripe)
- Blackberries
- Blueberries
- Granny Smith apples
- Grapefruits
- Lemons
- Limes
- Raspberries

LOW-FAT PROTEINS

Protein is required for the body's growth, maintenance, and repair. It is vital for almost every bodily process, including metabolism, digestion, and transportation. A major component of muscles, tissues, and organs, protein is needed to support a strong and healthy immune system. Just like healthy fats, protein helps keep you fuller longer and regulates blood sugar, both of which are essential for weight loss.

PROTEIN POWDER

A few recipes in this book contain protein powder. When shopping, look for a vegan (dairy-free) protein source and be sure to check labels to avoid powders with added sugar. If you do not want to use protein powder, simply substitute chia seeds, flaxseed, or shelled hemp seeds. The idea is to increase protein in each meal or snack to help keep you feeling fuller longer. Two brands I recommend are Sunwarrior Plant-Based Organic Protein and Garden of Life Raw Organic Meal Shake & Meal Replacement. The best dairy-free protein sources include hemp, which is a complete protein, and protein powders made from nuts, seeds, or pea protein.

Low-fat proteins include the following:

- Beans
- Chicken
- Chickpeas
- Eggs

- Fish
- Lean Beef
- Lentils
- Nuts

- Quinoa
- Seafood
- Seeds
- Turkey

Nutrition Tips

I want to empower you to make healthy choices throughout this detox and beyond with tips to help you eat in moderation as well as information on how to determine your own target calorie count.

EAT IN MODERATION

Here are some tips for eating in moderation:

1. Drink water throughout the day and before meals. It is one of the easiest ways to improve your health and energy level and to feel fuller. Aim to drink half of your body weight in ounces each day (so about 75 ounces for a 150-pound person).

2. Eat from a small plate or bowl. Large bowls and plates tend to lead to larger portions.

3. Slow down and practice mindful eating. When you quickly and mindlessly rush through your meal, you're not giving your brain and body a chance to feel satisfied.

4. Track what you're eating in your journal. Record what you eat and how you feel before and after eating. This record will help you become more aware of how much you should be eating and which foods make you feel good.

DETERMINE YOUR TARGET CALORIE INTAKE

One of the most challenging aspects of nutrition is determining your daily target calorie intake, which affects your metabolic rate. Our metabolism is like a fire—go too long without putting any wood on, and the flame burns out; stoke the fire with the right amount of wood, and a consistently hot burn results. We want to regularly fuel our bodies with healthy food to keep our metabolism revved up.

Apps such as MyFitnessPal, Start Simple with MyPlate, Lose It!, and Lifesum can tell you how many calories you should consume after you plug in your age, weight, and goal (whether it be weight gain, loss, or maintenance). You can also calculate your caloric needs yourself by searching online for the equation, then plugging in your basal metabolic rate and your physical activity level.

Good Habits

These good habits will help you get the full benefit of your sugar detox:

1. Keep journaling about your goals and why they are important to help you keep motivated after your detox is completed.

2. Develop a solid morning routine to set up your day for success.

    - Wake up and drink one glass of lemon water with probiotics.
    - Journal gratitude statements or set an intention for the day.
    - Meditate, even if it's only for five minutes.
    - Move your body in a way that feels good that day.
    - Enjoy a nourishing breakfast.
    - Begin the workday.

3. Make daily movement and workouts a lifelong practice.

4. Meditate and make time for relaxation and self-care.

5. Continue to meal plan and prep. If you have healthy food available consistently, you will make better choices.

6. Make sleep a priority. Sleep deprivation makes your body crave sugary foods, and you feel hungrier throughout the day.

Living a Low-Sugar Life

Once you complete your sugar detox, reintroduce foods slowly and one at a time to avoid stomach upset and a return to unhealthy habits. To keep your healthy efforts going, avoid processed and refined foods entirely. Stick to real, whole foods, slowly adding more fruits, dark chocolate, and grains. If you do not feel well after eating the foods that are reintroduced, consider eliminating them altogether.

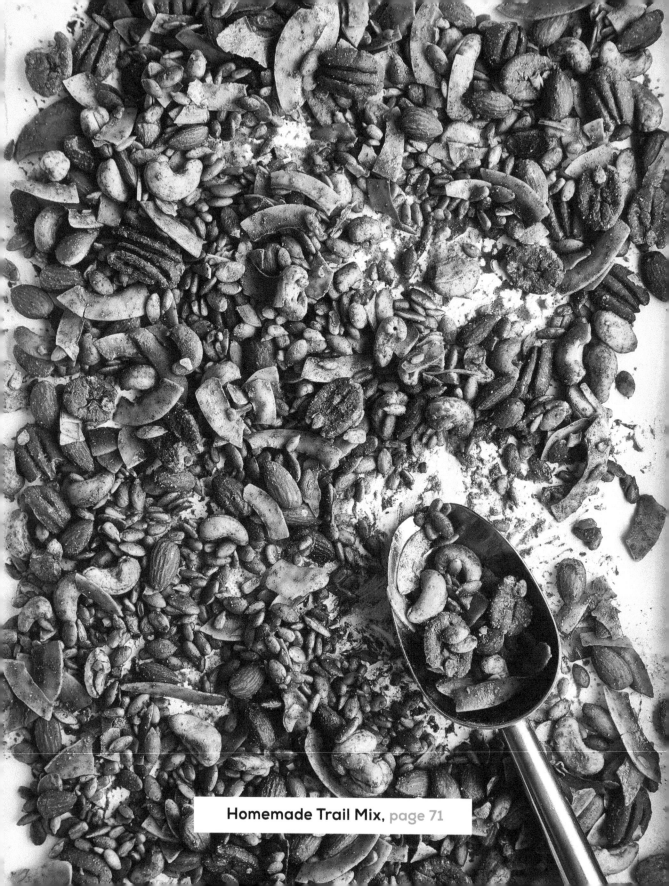

Homemade Trail Mix, page 71

3

Your 10-Day Sugar Detox Meal Plans

The following sugar detox meal plans reflect the way I prep and eat at home. Within the recipes you will see meal prep tips, recipe modifications, and ideas for leftovers, and each meal plan will be accompanied by a corresponding weekly shopping list; make sure to check your kitchen before you shop to see what you already have so you don't overstock on foods. This strategy keeps costs down, saves time in the store, and reduces food waste.

Select one of the four meal plans that best fits your current lifestyle and nutritional goals. Even if you are not much of a cook or have little to no experience cooking, you'll find it easy to cook lean meats, seafood, vegan meals, and detox staples like my Homemade Barbecue Sauce (page 80) or Cashew Cheese Sauce (page 84). Each recipe aims to educate you on the benefits of what you are eating so you understand exactly how you're nourishing your body from the inside out. Let's dig in!

LEAN MEAT MEAL PLAN

The Lean Meat Meal Plan is designed for anyone who consumes meat and animal proteins as part of their diet. The focus is on easy, nutrient-dense meals that are high in protein, healthy fats, and lots of vegetables. I recommend buying grass-fed, not grain-fed, lean meats, and organic is a big plus, too.

DAY	MEAL	RECIPE
DAY 1	Breakfast	Egg and Veggie Muffin Cups (1 to 2) 58
	Snack	½ cup sliced red bell pepper and ½ cup sliced cucumber with 2 tablespoons hummus
	Lunch	Apple and Almond Crunch Salad 91
	Dinner	Spinach and Feta Turkey Burger 159 with Roasted Veggie Mix 69
DAY 2	Breakfast	Green Goddess Smoothie 62
	Snack	Leftover Egg and Veggie Muffin Cups (1 to 2)
	Lunch	Leftover Spinach and Feta Turkey Burger with leftover Apple and Almond Crunch Salad
	Dinner	Zoodle Beef Chow Mein 158
DAY 3	Breakfast	Sweet Potato Toast 52
	Snack	½ cup sliced red bell pepper and ½ cup sliced cucumber with 2 tablespoons hummus, or 2 leftover Egg and Veggie Muffin Cups
	Lunch	Leftover Zoodle Beef Chow Mein
	Dinner	Peanut Chicken Tacos in Lettuce Wraps 162

LEAN MEAT MEAL PLAN CONTINUED

DAY	MEAL	RECIPE
DAY 4	Breakfast	Coconut Chia Porridge **49**
	Snack	Homemade Trail Mix (¼ cup) **71**
	Lunch	Leftover Peanut Chicken Tacos in Lettuce Wraps
	Dinner	Blackened White Fish **143** with mixed greens salad
DAY 5	Breakfast	Green Matcha Smoothie **63**
	Snack	Leftover Homemade Trail Mix (¼ cup)
	Lunch	Leftover Blackened White Fish with mixed greens salad
	Dinner	Chicken and Veggie Kabobs **157**
DAY 6	Breakfast	Healthy Breakfast Sausage Cakes **53** with Sweet Potato Toast **52**
	Snack	Roasted Veggie Mix **69** with hummus
	Lunch	Leftover Chicken and Veggie Kabobs over mixed greens
	Dinner	Slow Cooker Thai-Inspired Coconut Curry Chickpea Soup **106**

LEAN MEAT MEAL PLAN CONTINUED

DAY	MEAL	RECIPE
DAY 7	Breakfast	Leftover Healthy Breakfast Sausage Cakes
	Snack	Chipotle Barbecue Roasted Chickpeas 70 and leftover Roasted Veggie Mix
	Lunch	Leftover Slow Cooker Thai-Inspired Coconut Curry Chickpea Soup
	Dinner	Cashew Chicken with Cauliflower Rice 150
DAY 8	Breakfast	Blueberry Protein Pancakes (1 to 2) 55
	Snack	Super Seed Crackers 68 with 2 tablespoons hummus
	Lunch	Leftover Cashew Chicken with Cauliflower Rice
	Dinner	Almond-Crusted Salmon 138 with mixed greens salad
DAY 9	Breakfast	Chocolate Chia Pudding 48
	Snack	Leftover Seed Crackers with 2 tablespoons hummus and ½ cup sliced red bell pepper
	Lunch	Garlic Shrimp Zoodles 145
	Dinner	Southwest Turkey Chili 168
DAY 10	Breakfast	Chocolate Dream Smoothie 65
	Snack	1 Banana Bread Quinoa Bar 180
	Lunch	Leftover Southwest Turkey Chili
	Dinner	Chicken Detox Stew 96

PANTRY LIST, DAYS 1 TO 10

BEANS, LEGUMES, AND NUTS

- ½ cup almond flour
- ¼ cup almonds
- 1 (15-ounce) can black beans
- ¾ cup cashews
- 1 (15.5-ounce) can chickpeas
- 1 jar all-natural peanut or almond butter
- ¼ cup peanuts
- ¼ cup pecans
- ¼ cup pine nuts

CANNED AND PACKAGED GOODS

- ¼ cup unsweetened applesauce
- 4 quarts broth (vegetable, chicken, or beef)
- ½ cup unsweetened coconut flakes
- 2 (13.5-ounce) cans coconut milk
- 1 jar red curry paste
- Frank's RedHot Original sauce
- 1 (4-ounce) can diced green chiles (optional)
- Nutritional yeast
- Tamari or coconut aminos
- 1 (28-ounce) can diced tomatoes
- Pure vanilla extract

GRAINS AND POWDERS

- Baking powder
- Baking soda
- ½ cup gluten-free bread crumbs
- Cacao powder
- Chlorella powder (optional)
- Green matcha powder
- 1 cup gluten-free rolled oats
- 1 cup vegan chocolate protein powder
- ¾ cup vegan vanilla protein powder
- ½ cup quinoa
- Tapioca starch (optional)

OILS AND VINEGARS

- Avocado oil
- Balsamic vinegar
- Coconut oil
- Olive oil
- Rice vinegar
- Toasted sesame oil

SEEDS

- ¼ cup chia seeds
- 1 cup ground flaxseed
- 1 cup shelled hemp seeds
- 1 cup pumpkin seeds
- ½ cup sesame seeds
- ¼ cup sunflower seeds

HERBS AND SPICES, DAYS 1 TO 10

- Freshly ground black pepper
- Cayenne
- Chili powder
- Ground cinnamon
- Ground cumin
- Yellow curry powder
- Garlic salt
- Ground ginger
- Onion powder
- Paprika
- Dried parsley
- Poultry seasoning
- Pumpkin pie spice
- Salt
- Dried thyme
- Ground turmeric

PERISHABLES, DAYS 1 TO 5

REFRIGERATED ITEMS

- Half gallon unsweetened original almond milk
- 11 eggs
- ¾ cup egg whites
- 4 ounces feta cheese (optional)
- 1 (8-ounce) container hummus

MEAT AND SEAFOOD

- 8 boneless, skinless chicken breasts
- 1 (8-ounce) flank steak
- 1 pound lean ground turkey
- 2 to 4 wild-caught white fish fillets

PRODUCE

- 1 green apple
- 16 ounces arugula
- 2 avocados
- 1 beet
- 1 orange bell pepper
- 4 red bell peppers
- 1 yellow bell pepper
- 1 head red cabbage
- 5 medium carrots
- 1 head cauliflower
- 1 bunch fresh cilantro
- 2 English cucumbers
- 9 garlic cloves
- 1 inch fresh ginger
- 2 lemons
- 1 head iceberg lettuce
- 1 lime
- 2 (8-ounce) packages cremini mushrooms
- 1 red onion
- 3 yellow onions
- 1 scallion
- ¼ cup snap peas (optional)
- 12 ounces spinach
- 1 pint cherry tomatoes
- 3 cups zoodles, or 2 zucchinis to spiralize

PERISHABLES, DAYS 6 TO 10

REFRIGERATED ITEMS

- Half gallon unsweetened original almond milk
- 1 egg
- 1 (8-ounce) container hummus

MEAT AND SEAFOOD

- 6 boneless, skinless chicken breasts
- 2 pounds boneless, skinless chicken thighs
- 2 (5-ounce) wild-caught salmon fillets
- 30 frozen deveined shrimp
- 1 pound lean ground turkey

PRODUCE

- 10 green apples
- 3 bananas
- 1 green bell pepper
- 1 orange bell pepper
- 5 red bell peppers
- 2 heads broccoli
- 4 medium carrots
- 1 green cabbage
- 1 red cabbage
- 1 head cauliflower plus 2 cups cauliflower rice (or an extra 2 heads cauliflower)
- 1 bunch fresh cilantro
- 1 English cucumber
- 15 garlic cloves
- 2 inches fresh ginger
- 1 lemon
- 1 piece lemongrass (optional)
- 1 (24-ounce) package mixed greens
- 3 yellow onions
- 1 (24-ounce) package spinach
- 1 sweet potato
- 3 cups zoodles, or 2 zucchinis to spiralize

PESCATARIAN MEAL PLAN

The Pescatarian Meal Plan is designed for anyone who follows a diet that includes fish, dairy, and eggs but no meat. This is a largely plant-based meal plan including vegetarian dishes as well as seafood dishes. The focus is on nutrient-dense, real whole foods; lean proteins; and healthy fats. If you are looking to transition to a more plant-based lifestyle but still love fish and other seafood, this meal plan will work wonderfully for you.

DAY	MEAL	RECIPE
DAY 1	Breakfast	Chocolate Chia Pudding **48**
	Snack	Super Seed Crackers **68** with 2 tablespoons hummus
	Lunch	Arugula and Quinoa Salad **90**
	Dinner	Almond-Crusted Salmon **138** with mixed greens salad
DAY 2	Breakfast	Salmon Cake with Roasted Red Pepper Drizzle **142** and Sweet Potato Toast **52**
	Snack	Super Seed Crackers **68** with hummus and ½ cup sliced red bell pepper
	Lunch	Leftover Almond-Crusted Salmon with mixed greens salad
	Dinner	Greek Burger **118** with Roasted Veggie Mix **69**

PESCATARIAN MEAL PLAN CONTINUED

DAY	MEAL	RECIPE
DAY 3	Breakfast	Leftover Salmon Cake and leftover Sweet Potato Toast
	Snack	Green Matcha Smoothie 63
	Lunch	Leftover Greek Burger with mixed greens salad
	Dinner	Blackened White Fish 143 with Roasted Veggie Mix 69
DAY 4	Breakfast	Green Goddess Smoothie 62
	Snack	Super Seed Crackers 68 with 2 tablespoons hummus (can add raw veggies such as cucumber and celery)
	Lunch	Leftover Blackened Fish with leftover Roasted Veggie Mix
	Dinner	Shrimp Buddha Bowl 136
DAY 5	Breakfast	Immune-Boosting Smoothie 64
	Snack	Chipotle Barbecue Roasted Chickpeas 70
	Lunch	Split Pea and Pumpkin Soup 97
	Dinner	Mushroom Stroganoff with Garlic Cauliflower Mash 122

PESCATARIAN MEAL PLAN CONTINUED

DAY	MEAL	RECIPE
DAY 6	Breakfast	Blueberry Protein Pancakes (1 to 2) **55**
	Snack	Leftover Chipotle Barbecue Roasted Chickpeas
	Lunch	Leftover Mushroom Stroganoff with Garlic Cauliflower Mash
	Dinner	Cajun White Fish **147** with mixed greens salad
DAY 7	Breakfast	Egg and Veggie Muffin Cups (1 to 2) or Sweet Potato Toast **52**
	Snack	Leftover Blueberry Protein Pancakes (1 to 2)
	Lunch	Leftover Split Pea and Pumpkin Soup
	Dinner	Moroccan-Spiced Chickpea Bowl **126**
DAY 8	Breakfast	Leftover Egg and Veggie Muffin Cups (1 to 2) or leftover Sweet Potato Toast
	Snack	½ cup sliced red bell pepper and ½ cup sliced cucumber with 2 tablespoons hummus
	Lunch	Leftover Moroccan-Spiced Chickpea Bowl
	Dinner	Garlic Shrimp Zoodles **145**
DAY 9	Breakfast	Tofu Scramble Stir-Fry **57**
	Snack	Homemade Trail Mix (¼ cup) **71**
	Lunch	Leftover Garlic Shrimp Zoodles
	Dinner	Zoodle Lasagna with Basil Cashew Cheese **132**

PESCATARIAN MEAL PLAN CONTINUED

DAY	MEAL	RECIPE
DAY 10	Breakfast	Leftover Tofu Scramble Stir-Fry
	Snack	Leftover Homemade Trail Mix (¼ cup)
	Lunch	Leftover Zoodle Lasagna with Basil Cashew Cheese
	Dinner	Mushroom and Pesto Shrimp 140

PANTRY LIST, DAYS 1 TO 10

BEANS, LEGUMES, AND NUTS

- 1 jar all-natural almond or peanut butter
- ¾ cup almond flour
- ¼ cup almonds
- 1 (15-ounce) can black beans

- 3¾ cups cashews
- 3 (15.5-ounce) cans chickpeas (or 6 cups cooked)

- ¼ cup pecans
- ¼ cup pine nuts
- 2 cups dried yellow split peas

CANNED AND PACKAGED GOODS

- 1 jar black olives
- 8 quarts broth (vegetable, chicken or beef)
- ½ cup unsweetened coconut flakes
- Dijon mustard

- Frank's RedHot Original sauce
- Nutritional yeast
- 1 (16-ounce) can pumpkin purée
- 1 (12-ounce) jar roasted red peppers

- 2 (6-ounce) cans sockeye salmon
- Tamari or coconut aminos
- 2 (28-ounce) cans diced tomatoes
- Pure vanilla extract

GRAINS AND POWDERS

- Baking powder
- ⅓ cup gluten-free bread crumbs
- Chlorella powder (optional)
- Green matcha powder
- 1 cup gluten-free rolled oats
- 1½ cups vegan protein powder
- 2 cups quinoa

OILS AND VINEGARS

- Avocado oil
- Balsamic vinegar
- Coconut oil
- Olive oil
- Toasted sesame oil

SEEDS

- ¾ cup chia seeds
- ¾ cup ground flaxseed
- 1 cup shelled hemp seeds
- 1 cup pumpkin seeds
- ½ cup sesame seeds
- ¾ cup sunflower seeds

HERBS AND SPICES, DAYS 1 TO 10

- Freshly ground black pepper
- Cayenne
- Chili powder
- Ground cinnamon
- Ground coriander
- Ground cumin
- Garam masala
- Garlic powder
- Ground ginger
- Greek seasoning
- Onion powder
- Dried oregano
- Paprika
- Dried parsley
- Pumpkin pie spice
- Red pepper flakes
- Salt
- Dried thyme
- Ground turmeric

PERISHABLES, DAYS 1 TO 5

REFRIGERATED ITEMS

- Half gallon unsweetened original almond milk
- 3 eggs
- ¼ cup dairy-free feta cheese (optional)
- 1 container hummus

MEAT AND SEAFOOD

- 4 basa fish fillets, or any other white fish
- 4 salmon fillets
- 30 frozen deveined shrimp

PRODUCE

- 1 green apple
- 2 cups arugula
- 1 avocado
- 1 banana
- 1 beet
- 3 red bell peppers
- 1 to 2 heads broccoli
- 1 green cabbage
- 1 red cabbage
- 4 medium carrots
- 2 heads cauliflower, or 1 head cauliflower and 4 cups cauliflower rice
- 1 pint cherry tomatoes
- 1 bunch fresh cilantro
- 1 English cucumber
- 1 bunch fresh dill
- 12 garlic cloves
- 1 to 2 inches fresh ginger
- 1 grapefruit
- 1 cup kale (optional)
- 1 lemon
- 2 (8-ounce) containers cremini mushrooms
- 3 yellow onions
- 2 scallions
- 3 cups spinach
- 2 sweet potatoes
- 1 tomato

PERISHABLES, DAYS 6 TO 10

REFRIGERATED ITEMS

- Half gallon unsweetened original almond milk
- 9 eggs
- ¾ cup egg whites
- 1 (14-ounce) package extra-firm tofu

MEAT AND SEAFOOD

- 4 basa fillets (or any other white fish)
- 20 frozen deveined shrimp

PRODUCE

- 1 avocado
- 3 cups baby spinach
- 4 cups fresh basil
- 4 red bell peppers
- ¼ cup blueberries (fresh or frozen)
- 2 heads broccoli
- 1 red cabbage
- 2 heads cauliflower
- 19 garlic cloves
- 1 lemon
- 1 lime
- 1 (24-ounce) package mixed greens
- 3 (8-ounce) containers mushrooms
- 3 onions
- 2 sweet potatoes
- 1 tomato
- 4 zucchinis

VEGAN MEAL PLAN

The Vegan Meal Plan is for those who consume no animal products whatsoever (no meat, dairy, eggs, nada). The recipes are carefully selected to ensure you are getting adequate protein, healthy fats, and essential nutrients such as vitamin B_{12}, iron, and zinc. As with all the meal plans, the recipes were not only designed to be healthy; the big focus is to ensure they are delicious, too. Most sugar detox programs or weight loss plans fail to include meal plans based on people's lifestyle preferences. I am really proud to include this section as I truly believe in adopting a more plant-based lifestyle and I think there are a bunch of you out there who feel the same way.

DAY	MEAL	RECIPE
DAY 1	Breakfast	Green Goddess Smoothie 62
	Snack	Super Seed Crackers 68 with 2 tablespoons hummus
	Lunch	Arugula and Quinoa Salad 90
	Dinner	Mushroom Stroganoff with Garlic Cauliflower Mash 122
DAY 2	Breakfast	Coconut Chia Porridge 49
	Snack	Leftover Super Seed Crackers with 2 tablespoons hummus
	Lunch	Split Pea and Pumpkin Soup 97
	Dinner	Portobello Fajita Bowl 128

VEGAN MEAL PLAN CONTINUED

DAY	MEAL	RECIPE
DAY 3	Breakfast	Chocolate Chia Pudding 48
	Snack	Leftover Super Seed Crackers with 1 tablespoon hummus or sliced veggies and hummus
	Lunch	Leftover Split Pea and Pumpkin Soup
	Dinner	Peanut Chickpea Tacos in Lettuce Wraps 112
DAY 4	Breakfast	Leftover Chocolate Chia Pudding
	Snack	Roasted Veggie Mix 69
	Lunch	Leftover Peanut Chickpea Tacos in Lettuce Wraps
	Dinner	Black Bean Enchilada Bowl 124
DAY 5	Breakfast	Sweet Potato Toast 52
	Snack	Chipotle Barbecue Roasted Chickpeas 70
	Lunch	Leftover Black Bean Enchilada Bowl
	Dinner	Lentil Burrito Bowl 125
DAY 6	Breakfast	Baked Oatmeal 56
	Snack	Leftover Chipotle Barbecue Roasted Chickpeas or leftover Roasted Veggie Mix
	Lunch	Leftover Lentil Burrito Bowl
	Dinner	Moroccan-Spiced Chickpea Bowl 126

VEGAN MEAL PLAN CONTINUED

DAY	MEAL	RECIPE
DAY 7	Breakfast	Leftover Baked Oatmeal
	Snack	Homemade Trail Mix (¼ cup) **71**
	Lunch	Leftover Moroccan-Spiced Chickpea Bowl
	Dinner	Lentil and Mushroom Burgers **114** with Roasted Veggie Mix **69**
DAY 8	Breakfast	Chocolate Dream Smoothie **65**
	Snack	Leftover Trail Mix (¼ cup)
	Lunch	Leftover Lentil and Mushroom Burger over mixed greens
	Dinner	Slow Cooker Barbecue Lentil Chili **131**
DAY 9	Breakfast	Tofu Scramble Stir-Fry **57**
	Snack	1 green apple and 1 tablespoon almond butter
	Lunch	Leftover Slow Cooker Barbecue Lentil Chili
	Dinner	Thai-Inspired Red Curry with Cauliflower Rice **104**
DAY 10	Breakfast	Leftover Tofu Scramble Stir-Fry
	Snack	1 Banana Bread Quinoa Bar **180**
	Lunch	Leftover Thai-Inspired Red Curry with Cauliflower Rice
	Dinner	Lasagna-Stuffed Portobello Mushrooms **120**

PLAN PANTRY LIST, DAYS 1 TO 10

CANNED AND PACKAGED GOODS

- ¼ cup unsweetened applesauce
- 1 can 6-bean mix
- 3 (15.5-ounce) cans chickpeas
- ¼ cup unsweetened coconut flakes
- 2 (13.5 ounce) cans coconut milk
- 1 jar red curry paste
- Frank's RedHot Original sauce
- 2 cups dried brown lentils
- Nutritional yeast
- Tamari or coconut aminos
- 3 (28-ounce) cans diced tomatoes
- 1 (6-ounce) can tomato paste
- Pure vanilla extract
- 2 quarts vegetable broth

GRAINS AND POWDERS

- Baking powder
- Cacao powder
- 1 teaspoon chlorella powder (optional)
- 3 cups gluten-free rolled oats
- ¾ cup vegan chocolate protein powder
- ½ cup vegan vanilla protein powder
- 3½ cups quinoa

LEGUMES, NUTS, AND NUT BUTTERS

- 1 jar all-natural almond or peanut butter
- ¼ cup almonds
- 4¼ cups cashews
- 4 cups dried brown lentils
- 2 cups dried red lentils
- ½ cup peanuts
- ¼ cups pecans
- 2 cups dried yellow split peas

OILS AND VINEGARS

- Apple cider vinegar
- Avocado oil
- Balsamic vinegar
- Coconut oil
- Olive oil
- Rice vinegar
- Toasted sesame oil

SEEDS

- 1½ cup chia seeds
- 1 cup ground flaxseed
- 1 cup shelled hemp seeds
- ¾ cup pumpkin seeds
- ½ cup sesame seeds
- ¾ cup sunflower seeds

HERBS AND SPICES, DAYS 1 TO 10

- Chili powder
- Ground cinnamon
- Ground coriander
- Ground cumin
- Yellow curry powder
- Garam masala
- Garlic salt
- Ground ginger
- Italian seasoning
- Onion powder
- Dried oregano
- Paprika
- Dried parsley
- Pumpkin pie spices
- Ground turmeric

PERISHABLES, DAYS 1 TO 5

REFRIGERATED ITEMS

- Half gallon unsweetened original almond milk
- 1 (8-ounce) container hummus

PRODUCE

- 10 green apples
- 2 cups arugula
- 2 avocados
- 1 banana
- 1 beet
- 1 orange bell pepper
- 4 red bell peppers
- 1 yellow bell pepper
- 1 head broccoli
- 1 green cabbage
- 1 red cabbage
- 1 head cauliflower, plus 4 cups cauliflower rice
- 1 bunch fresh cilantro (optional)
- 1 English cucumber
- 15 garlic cloves
- ½ inch fresh ginger
- 1 lemon
- 2 heads romaine or iceberg lettuce
- 1 lime
- 3 (8-ounce) packages cremini mushrooms
- 4 to 6 portobello mushrooms
- 1 red onion
- 3 yellow onions
- 1 medium pumpkin
- 1 scallion
- 3 cups spinach
- 1 sweet potato
- 2 tomatoes
- 3 cups zoodles, or 2 zucchinis

PERISHABLES, DAYS 6 TO 10

REFRIGERATED ITEMS

- Half gallon unsweetened original almond milk
- 1 (8-ounce) container hummus
- 1 (14-ounce) container extra-firm tofu

PRODUCE

- 2 avocados
- 4 bananas
- 1 bunch fresh basil
- 3 red bell peppers
- 2 yellow bell peppers
- 1 head broccoli
- 1 green cabbage
- 1 red cabbage
- 1 head cauliflower, plus 2 cups cauliflower rice
- 2 medium carrots
- 1 bunch fresh cilantro
- 1 English cucumber
- 16 garlic cloves
- 1 inch fresh ginger
- 2 cups kale (optional)
- 1 lemon
- 1 head iceberg lettuce
- 1 lime
- 2 (8-ounce) packages cremini mushrooms
- 4 to 6 portobello mushrooms
- 6 yellow onions
- 5½ cups spinach
- 1 tomato

VEGETARIAN MEAL PLAN

Given that dairy is not allowed on this detox, the main difference between this book's vegan and vegetarian meal plans is the inclusion of eggs. And fear not, the vegan dishes in this meal plan are so delicious that you won't even miss the cheese!

DAY	MEAL	RECIPE
DAY 1	Breakfast	2 Egg and Veggie Muffin Cups 58
	Snack	Super Seed Crackers 68 with 2 tablespoons hummus
	Lunch	Arugula and Quinoa Salad 90
	Dinner	Mushroom Stroganoff with Garlic Cauliflower Mash 122
DAY 2	Breakfast	2 leftover Egg and Veggie Muffin Cups
	Snack	Leftover Super Seed Crackers with 2 tablespoons hummus
	Lunch	Split Pea and Pumpkin Soup 97
	Dinner	Vegan Taco Bowl 127
DAY 3	Breakfast	Green Goddess Smoothie 62
	Snack	Leftover Super Seed Crackers with 1 tablespoon hummus or sliced veggies and hummus
	Lunch	Leftover Split Pea and Pumpkin Soup
	Dinner	Buffalo Chickpea Tacos in Lettuce Wraps 117

VEGETARIAN MEAL PLAN CONTINUED

DAY	MEAL	RECIPE
DAY 4	Breakfast	Coconut Chia Porridge 49
	Snack	Roasted Veggie Mix 69
	Lunch	Leftover Buffalo Chickpea Tacos in Lettuce Wraps
	Dinner	Lentil Burrito Bowl 125
DAY 5	Breakfast	Sweet Potato Toast 52 with almond butter
	Snack	Chipotle Barbecue Roasted Chickpeas 70
	Lunch	Leftover Lentil Burrito Bowl
	Dinner	Greek Burger 118 with leftover Roasted Veggie Mix
DAY 6	Breakfast	Baked Oatmeal 56
	Snack	Leftover Chipotle Barbecue Roasted Chickpeas and leftover Roasted Veggie Mix
	Lunch	Leftover Greek Burger with leftover Roasted Veggie Mix
	Dinner	Chickpeas with Cauliflower Rice 108
DAY 7	Breakfast	Leftover Baked Oatmeal
	Snack	Homemade Trail Mix (¼ cup) 71
	Lunch	Leftover Chickpeas with Cauliflower Rice
	Dinner	Slow Cooker Barbecue Lentil Chili 131

VEGETARIAN MEAL PLAN CONTINUED

DAY	MEAL	RECIPE
DAY 8	Breakfast	Chocolate Dream Smoothie **65**
	Snack	Leftover Homemade Trail Mix (¼ cup)
	Lunch	Leftover Barbecue Lentil Chili
	Dinner	Mexican-Inspired Stuffed Peppers **116**
DAY 9	Breakfast	Tofu Scramble Stir-Fry **57**
	Snack	1 green apple and 1 tablespoon almond butter
	Lunch	Leftover Mexican-Inspired Stuffed Peppers
	Dinner	Moroccan-Spiced Chickpea Bowl **126**
DAY 10	Breakfast	Leftover Tofu Scramble Stir-Fry
	Snack	Leftover Homemade Trail Mix (¼ cup)
	Lunch	Leftover Moroccan-Spiced Chickpea Bowl
	Dinner	Vegan Shepherd's Pie with Cauliflower Mash **130**

PANTRY LIST, DAYS 1 TO 10

BEANS, LEGUMES, AND NUTS

- ¼ cup almonds
- 1 jar all-natural almond butter
- 1 (16-ounce) package 6-bean mix
- ¾ cup cashews
- 16 ounces dried red lentils
- 2 cups dried yellow split peas
- ¼ cup pecans
- ½ cup chopped walnuts

CANNED AND PACKAGED GOODS

- 2 (15-ounce) can black beans
- 6 (15.5-ounce) cans chickpeas
- 1 (4-ounce) can diced green chiles (optional)
- ¾ cup unsweetened coconut flakes
- 1 (13.5-ounce) can coconut milk
- Frank's RedHot Original sauce
- Nutritional yeast
- 1 jar black pitted olives
- 1 jar roasted red peppers
- Tamari or coconut aminos
- 1 (14.5-ounce) can crushed tomatoes
- 3 (28-ounce) cans diced tomatoes
- 1 (6-ounce) can tomato paste
- Pure vanilla extract
- 4 quarts vegetable broth

GRAINS AND POWDERS

- ⅓ cup gluten-free bread crumbs
- 1 cup brown rice
- Cacao powder
- 3 cups gluten-free rolled oats
- ¼ cup vegan chocolate protein powder
- ½ cup vegan vanilla protein powder
- ½ cup quinoa

OILS AND VINEGARS

- Apple cider vinegar
- Avocado oil
- Balsamic vinegar
- Coconut oil
- Olive oil
- Toasted sesame oil

SEEDS

- ¼ cup chia seeds
- ¾ cup ground flaxseed
- ¾ cup shelled hemp seeds
- ¼ cup pumpkin seeds
- ½ cup sesame seeds
- ¾ cup sunflower seeds

HERBS AND SPICE, DAYS 1 TO 10

- Freshly ground black pepper
- Chili powder
- Ground chipotle chile
- Ground cinnamon
- Ground coriander
- Ground cumin
- Yellow curry powder
- Garam masala
- Garlic powder
- Ground ginger
- Greek seasoning
- Onion powder
- Dried oregano
- Paprika
- Pumpkin pie spice
- Salt
- Ground turmeric

PERISHABLES, DAYS 1 TO 5

REFRIGERATED ITEMS

- Half gallon unsweetened original almond milk
- Vegan butter or ghee
- 8 eggs
- ¾ cup egg whites
- ¼ cup feta cheese (optional)
- 1 (8-ounce) container hummus

PRODUCE

- 4 cups arugula or mixed greens
- 3 avocados
- 1 banana
- 1 beet
- 1 orange bell pepper
- 4 red bell peppers
- 4 cups broccoli florets
- 2 cups green cabbage
- 2 cups red cabbage
- 4 cups cauliflower rice, plus 2 cups cauliflower florets
- 1 bunch fresh cilantro
- 1 cucumber
- 1 bunch fresh dill
- 7 garlic cloves
- fresh ginger
- 1 head iceberg lettuce
- 1 head romaine lettuce
- 3 (8-ounce) containers cremini mushrooms
- 1 red onion
- 3 yellow onions
- 1 (16-ounce) can pumpkin purée
- 1 bunch scallions
- 1 (24-ounce) package spinach
- 1 sweet potato
- 3 tomatoes

PERISHABLES, DAYS 6 TO 10

REFRIGERATED ITEMS

- Half gallon unsweetened original almond milk
- 1 (8-ounce) container hummus
- 1 (14-ounce) container extra-firm tofu

PRODUCE

- 10 green apples
- 1 avocado
- 2 bananas
- 6 red bell peppers
- 1 yellow bell pepper
- 4 cups broccoli
- 2 cups green cabbage
- 2 cups red cabbage
- 4 cups cauliflower plus 4 cups cauliflower rice
- 1 bunch fresh cilantro
- 16 garlic cloves
- 1 inch fresh ginger
- 2 (8-ounce) packages cremini mushrooms
- 6 yellow onions
- 2 cups green peas
- 1 (24-ounce) package spinach
- 1 tomato

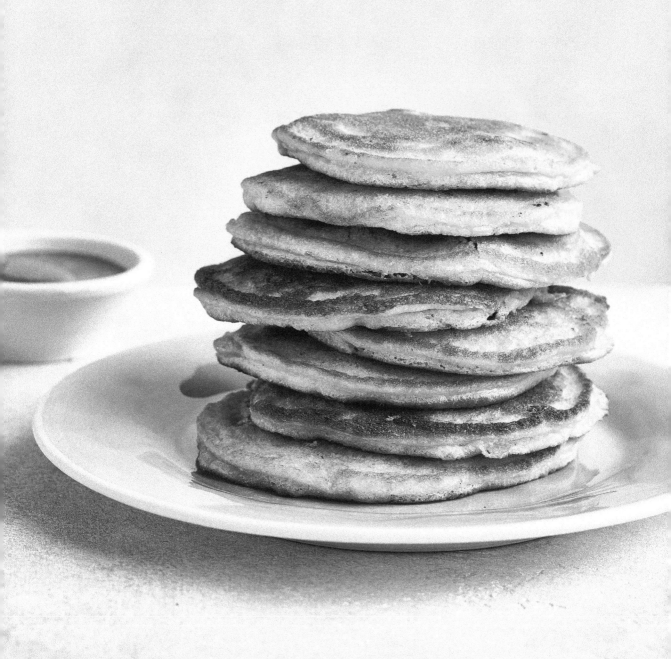

Blueberry Protein Pancakes, page 55

4

Breakfast

If you are not a morning person, one of the best ways to be sure to get a healthy breakfast is to prep the night before. Check out the Chocolate Chia Pudding (page 48) and Coconut Chia Porridge (page 49)—both can be made ahead of time and stored in glass jars for an easy grab-and-go breakfast. Similarly, the sausage cakes and oat bread recipes can be made ahead of time. Try doubling the protein pancake and egg cup recipes, which you can prep and freeze. Whichever meal you pick, your body will thank you. If you are not much of a food person in the morning, check out the next chapter to see the wide variety of smoothies.

Chocolate Chia Pudding

MAKES: 2–3 SERVINGS / **PREP TIME:**
10 MINUTES, PLUS OVERNIGHT TO CHILL

GLUTEN-FREE, VEGAN

Chia seeds are high in protein and rich in omega-3 fatty acids, which help reduce inflammation. These super seeds are also high in magnesium, potassium, calcium, iron, and fiber, all of which help sustain energy and maintain fullness.

2 cups unsweetened original almond milk

2 tablespoons cacao powder

2 tablespoons vegan chocolate protein powder or additional cacao powder (optional)

½ cup chia seeds

1 tablespoon almond butter

1 teaspoon pure vanilla extract

Blueberries, for topping (optional)

Unsweetened coconut flakes, for topping (optional)

1. In a large bowl, whisk together the almond milk, cacao powder, and chocolate protein powder (if using) until well combined, with no clumps.
2. Add the chia seeds, almond butter, and vanilla and whisk to combine.
3. Store in a container with a lid and refrigerate overnight.
4. In the morning, whisk again to break up any clumps. Place the mixture in a jar or bowl and top with blueberries or coconut flakes, if desired.

VARIATION TIP: If you want to sweeten this up naturally, add half a sliced banana.

PER SERVING Calories: 517; Saturated Fat: 5g; Total Fat: 32g; Protein: 29g; Total Carbs: 39g; Fiber: 29g; Sodium: 411mg

Coconut Chia Porridge

MAKES: 1 SERVING / **PREP TIME:** 10 MINUTES

GLUTEN-FREE, VEGAN

This recipe can be made in a mason jar. Sprinkle, pour, shake, and enjoy. For a little natural sweetness, try topping the porridge with 1 tablespoon of almond butter.

½ cup gluten-free rolled oats

¼ cup vegan vanilla protein powder

¼ cup unsweetened coconut flakes

3 tablespoons chia seeds

1 tablespoon pumpkin seeds

1 teaspoon pure vanilla extract

1 teaspoon ground cinnamon

¾ cup unsweetened vanilla almond milk

In a mason jar, put the oats, vanilla protein powder, coconut flakes, chia seeds, pumpkin seeds, vanilla, cinnamon, and almond milk. Cover and shake to combine. Let sit for 5 minutes, then stir and enjoy.

VARIATION TIP: You can also enjoy this dish warm! In a small pot over medium-low heat, cook the almond milk, oats, vanilla protein powder, coconut flakes, chia seeds, pumpkin seeds, vanilla, and cinnamon for 3 to 5 minutes until warm throughout.

PER SERVING Calories: 691; Saturated Fat: 10g; Total Fat: 32g; Protein: 42g; Total Carbs: 60g; Fiber: 24g; Sodium: 394mg

Savory Turkey Breakfast Skillet

MAKES: 4-5 SERVINGS / **PREP TIME:** 10 MINUTES / **COOK TIME:** 30 MINUTES

NUT-FREE

This breakfast skillet is as comforting as it is satisfying. The recipe can be enjoyed as is, but feel free to add eggs for some extra protein and top with Cashew Cheese Sauce (page 84).

1 sweet potato, cubed

1 or 2 cups Brussels sprouts, trimmed

2 tablespoons avocado oil, divided

Salt

Freshly ground black pepper

½ yellow onion, diced

3 garlic cloves, minced

1. Preheat the oven to 375°F and line a baking sheet with parchment paper.
2. Place the cubed sweet potatoes and Brussels sprouts on the baking sheet and drizzle with 1 tablespoon of avocado oil. Mix well to ensure everything is evenly coated and sprinkle with salt and pepper. Bake for 30 minutes, flipping halfway through, or until the sweet potatoes are fork-tender and the Brussels sprouts are golden.
3. Meanwhile, in a large skillet, heat the remaining 1 tablespoon of avocado oil over medium heat. Add the onion, garlic, mushrooms, and red pepper. Sauté for about 5 minutes, until the onion is translucent.

1 cup cremini mushrooms, chopped

1 red bell pepper, diced

1 pound lean ground turkey

1 tablespoon finely chopped fresh rosemary

1 teaspoon dried oregano

1 teaspoon garlic salt

½ teaspoon finely chopped fresh basil

½ teaspoon finely chopped fresh thyme

4. Add the turkey and cook until cooked through, stirring occasionally, about 10 minutes.
5. Once the turkey is cooked, add the rosemary, oregano, garlic salt, basil, and thyme to the meat mixture and stir.
6. Once the sweet potatoes and Brussels sprouts are done, add them to the meat mixture in the skillet and mix to incorporate.

SUBSTITUTION TIP: If you're not a fan of the spice mixture, substitute a Cajun spice mix and add black beans and diced tomatoes.

PER SERVING Calories: 258; Saturated Fat: 3g; Total Fat: 12g; Protein: 25g; Total Carbs: 15g; Fiber: 3g; Sodium: 112mg

Sweet Potato Toast

MAKES: 1 SERVING / **PREP TIME:** 5 MINUTES / **COOK TIME:** 15 MINUTES

GLUTEN-FREE, NUT-FREE, VEGETARIAN

Sweet potatoes are loaded with beta carotene, which gets converted to vitamin A, vitamin B$_6$, magnesium, and potassium. These tubers also contain both soluble and insoluble fiber, so you'll feel fuller longer. Choose your favorite way to serve them: Almond butter would also be a delicious protein add-on if you'd prefer that to the egg.

1 sweet potato

1 tablespoon avocado oil

1 egg

½ avocado, mashed

½ tomato, diced

1 scallion, chopped

1. Slice the sweet potato into thin bread-like pieces and place the two largest pieces in the toaster. Toast for 1 to 4 minutes, until soft and golden.
2. In a medium nonstick skillet, heat the avocado oil over medium heat. Crack the egg into the pan and lower the heat to slowly cook the whites, about 5 minutes. When the whites are completely set and the yolks begin to thicken, slide the spatula under the egg and gently flip. Cook the second side for 5 minutes, or to desired doneness.
3. To serve, place the toast on a plate and top with the egg, avocado, tomato, and scallion.

VARIATION TIP: Top with Cashew Cheese Sauce (page 84) or, for a sweeter version, top with almond butter and shelled hemp seeds.

PER SERVING Calories: 335; Saturated Fat: 3g; Total Fat: 18g; Protein: 10g; Total Carbs: 38g; Fiber: 11g; Sodium: 145mg

Healthy Breakfast Sausage Cakes

MAKES: 5 CAKES / PREP TIME: 10 MINUTES / COOK TIME: 10 MINUTES

GLUTEN-FREE, NUT-FREE

Enjoy this recipe with Sweet Potato Toast (page 52) or egg and avocado. It's simple enough to prep the sausage cakes and individually wrap and freeze them so you have a breakfast you can pull out to cook when you find yourself short on time.

1 teaspoon poultry seasoning

1 teaspoon onion powder

½ teaspoon garlic salt

½ teaspoon dried thyme

¼ teaspoon paprika

1 pound lean ground turkey

1 tablespoon avocado oil

1. In a small bowl, combine the poultry seasoning, onion powder, garlic salt, thyme, and paprika.
2. In a large bowl, combine the turkey and spice mixture. Mix with your hands and form into 5 patties.
3. In a large skillet, heat the avocado oil over medium heat. Add the sausage cakes and cook for 3 to 4 minutes per side, or until the meat is cooked through. Serve warm.

STORAGE TIP: Any uncooked sausage cakes will keep for up to one month in the freezer.
VARIATION TIP: Top with one egg or serve with Sweet Potato Toast (page 52).

PER SERVING Calories: 208; Saturated Fat: 3g; Total Fat: 12g; Protein: 22g; Total Carbs: 1g; Fiber: 0g; Sodium: 82mg

Oat Bread

MAKES: 4-6 SERVINGS / **PREP TIME:** 10 MINUTES / **COOK TIME:** 25 MINUTES

GLUTEN-FREE, VEGAN

This low-sugar gluten-free bread is delicious with almond butter.

½ cup almond flour

½ cup gluten-free rolled oats

¼ cup ground flaxseed

¼ cup hemp seeds

1 tablespoon chia seeds

½ teaspoon garlic powder

½ teaspoon salt

¼ teaspoon baking powder

1 cup unsweetened original almond milk

1 to 2 tablespoons pumpkin seeds

1. Preheat the oven to 375°F. Line a 9-by-9-inch casserole dish with parchment paper.
2. In a large bowl, combine the flour, oats, flaxseed, hemp seeds, chia seeds, garlic powder, salt, and baking powder.
3. Add the almond milk and stir. Let sit for 10 minutes, then pour the batter into the casserole dish. Evenly spread the mixture and sprinkle the top with the pumpkin seeds.
4. Bake for 20 to 25 minutes, until the bread is firm and the top is golden. Allow to cool for 5 minutes and serve.

SUBSTITUTION TIP: If you want to make this recipe nut-free, replace the almond flour with oat flour and the almond milk with unsweetened coconut milk or water.

PER SERVING Calories: 254; Saturated Fat: 1g; Total Fat: 17g; Protein: 10g; Total Carbs: 15g; Fiber: 7g; Sodium: 386mg

Blueberry Protein Pancakes

MAKES: 3 SERVINGS / **PREP TIME:** 10 MINUTES / **COOK TIME:** 10 MINUTES

GLUTEN-FREE, VEGETARIAN

Vanilla protein powder makes these pancakes exceptionally satisfying. Eat them as is or add 2 tablespoons of raw cacao powder for a chocolate twist.

½ cup vegan vanilla protein powder

¼ cup almond flour or gluten-free whole-wheat flour

1 teaspoon baking powder

1 egg

¼ cup unsweetened vanilla almond milk

¼ cup frozen blueberries

½ tablespoon avocado or coconut oil

Apple Butter (page 86; optional)

Cashew Fruit Dip (page 79; optional)

1 tablespoon almond butter (optional)

1. In a large bowl, combine the protein powder, flour, and baking powder.
2. Add the egg, almond milk, and blueberries and stir until just incorporated.
3. In a large skillet, heat the oil over medium heat. Pour in ¼ cup of the batter for each pancake. Cook for 1 to 3 minutes, or until bubbles start to appear on top of the pancake. Flip and cook for 2 to 3 minutes more, until cooked through and golden on the outside.
4. If using, top with the homemade apple butter, cashew fruit dip, or almond butter, and serve warm.

SUBSTITUTION TIP: Make this recipe vegan by omitting the egg and instead combining 3 tablespoons of ground flaxseed and ⅓ cup of water in a small bowl. Stir and let sit for 10 minutes until the mixture thickens to an egg-like consistency.

PER SERVING Calories: 143; Saturated Fat: 1g; Total Fat: 7g; Protein: 17g; Total Carbs: 4g; Fiber: 1g; Sodium: 180mg

Baked Oatmeal

MAKES: 4–6 SERVINGS / **PREP TIME:** 5 MINUTES, PLUS
30 MINUTES TO CHILL / **COOK TIME:** 25 MINUTES

GLUTEN-FREE, VEGAN

Enjoy this recipe as is or switch it up by substituting 1 banana for ⅓ cup of pumpkin purée (do not use pumpkin pie filling, which has added sugar). If you want to make it a little bit sweeter, add 1 to 2 tablespoons of Apple Butter (page 86).

1 banana

3½ cups unsweetened original almond milk

2 cups gluten-free rolled oats

½ cup vegan vanilla or chocolate protein powder

½ cup chia seeds

1 teaspoon ground cinnamon

1 teaspoon vanilla

1. Preheat the oven to 350°F. Line a 9-by-9-inch casserole dish with parchment paper.
2. In a large bowl, mash the banana until smooth. Stir in the almond milk, oats, protein powder, chia seeds, cinnamon, and vanilla until well combined. Cover and refrigerate for 30 minutes.
3. Once the mixture is chilled, scoop it onto a baking sheet and flatten it out with a spatula.
4. Bake for 25 minutes, until firm. Slice into bars and serve warm.

VARIATION TIP: This recipe can be modified with these optional toppings: a diced apple coated in cinnamon, almonds, blueberries, pecans, pumpkin seeds, or walnuts.

PER SERVING Calories: 442; Saturated Fat: 1g; Total Fat: 17g; Protein: 23g; Total Carbs: 49g; Fiber: 17g; Sodium: 428mg

Tofu Scramble Stir-Fry

MAKES: 2–3 SERVINGS / PREP TIME: 10 MINUTES / COOK TIME: 15 MINUTES

GLUTEN-FREE, NUT-FREE, VEGAN

This recipe is tailored to vegans and vegetarians. Tofu is a great source of protein, and nutritional yeast is an excellent source of vitamin B_{12}, which typically comes from animal-based products. Nutritional yeast is inactive yeast that gives food a cheesy flavor and that can be sprinkled over salads and bowls or added to dressings. My favorite brands are Bob's Red Mill or Bragg. Cashew Cheese Sauce (page 84) is a great topping for this recipe.

1 tablespoon avocado oil

¼ yellow onion, diced

2 garlic cloves, minced

1 (8-ounce) package cremini mushrooms, sliced

1 red bell pepper, diced

1 to 2 cups spinach

4 to 6 tablespoons nutritional yeast

1 teaspoon ground turmeric

Salt

Freshly ground black pepper

1 (14-ounce) package firm tofu, crumbled

1. In a large skillet, heat the avocado oil over medium heat. Sauté the onion, garlic, and mushrooms for 5 to 7 minutes, until the onion is translucent and softened. Add the red pepper and sauté for another 3 minutes, until fork-tender. Stir in the spinach, nutritional yeast, and turmeric and season with salt and pepper.
2. Crumble the tofu into the mixture and reduce the heat. Stir to combine and cook for another 5 to 10 minutes, until the entire mixture is cooked through.
3. Serve warm.

VARIATION TIP: Top with diced tomatoes, avocados, or my Cashew Cheese Sauce (page 84).

PER SERVING Calories: 348; Saturated Fat: 3g; Total Fat: 17g; Protein: 31g; Total Carbs: 26g; Fiber: 10g; Sodium: 634mg

Egg and Veggie Muffin Cups

MAKES: 12 SERVINGS / **PREP TIME:** 10 MINUTES / **COOK TIME:** 25 MINUTES

GLUTEN-FREE, NUT-FREE, VEGETARIAN

Customize this recipe by adding your favorite veggies, cooked meat, and dairy-free feta or goat cheese. This recipe is freezer friendly. You can reheat it in the oven or microwave or on the stovetop. These cups taste good cold, too.

1 tablespoon avocado oil

¼ yellow onion, diced

1 cup cremini mushrooms, finely chopped

1 red bell pepper, diced

1 garlic clove, minced

1 cup baby spinach

6 whole eggs plus 6 additional egg whites

Tomatoes, diced, for topping (optional)

Scallions, chopped, for topping (optional)

Avocado, diced, for topping (optional)

1. Preheat the oven to 350°F. Fill a muffin tin with liners.
2. In a large skillet, heat the avocado oil over medium heat. Sauté the onion, mushrooms, red pepper, and garlic for 5 to 7 minutes, until the onion is almost translucent. Add the spinach and cook until the spinach is wilted.
3. In a medium bowl, add the whole eggs and egg whites. Whisk until combined.
4. Divide the veggie mixture evenly among the muffin cups, then pour the egg mixture over the veggies until each cup is three-quarters full. Bake for 15 to 20 minutes, until firm.
5. Serve as is, or, if using, top with one or more of the tomatoes, scallions, or avocado.

STORAGE TIP: For an easy breakfast or snack you can heat up in no time, double the recipe and store individual cups in an airtight container in the freezer for up to one month.

PER SERVING Calories: 67; Saturated Fat: 1g; Total Fat: 4g; Protein: 6g; Total Carbs: 2g; Fiber: 0g; Sodium: 59mg

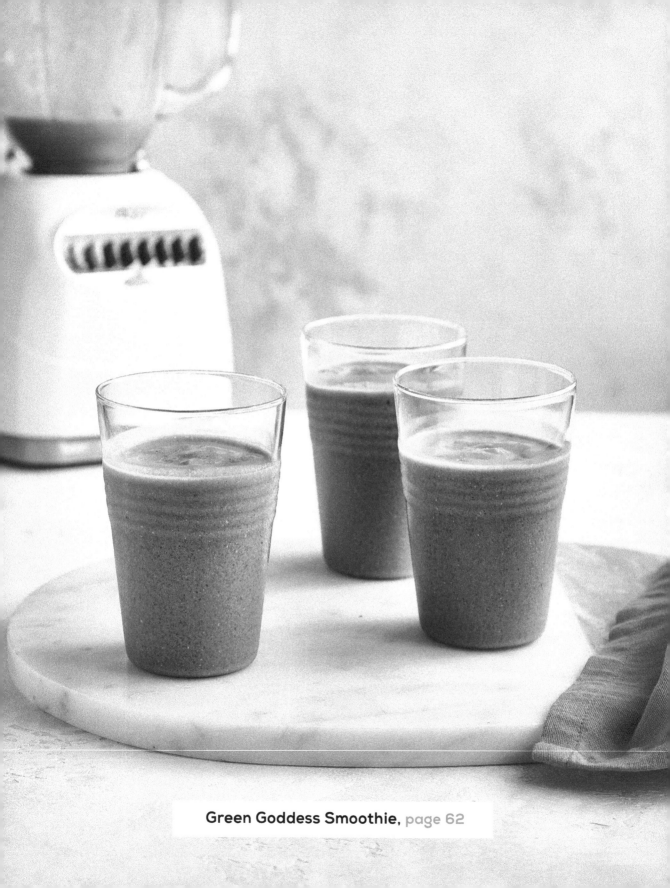

Green Goddess Smoothie, page 62

5

Smoothies
and Snacks

This chapter contains five awesome smoothie recipes that take less than 5 minutes to make and that include a variety of essential vitamins, minerals, phytonutrients, fiber, protein, and healthy fats.

The Super Seed Crackers (page 68) and Homemade Trail Mix (page 71) contain protein and fat that will keep you feeling fuller longer. They can be prepped at the beginning of the week. The Roasted Veggie Mix (page 69) and Chipotle Barbecue Roasted Chickpeas (page 70) are alternatives to raw veggies and hummus.

Green Goddess Smoothie

MAKES: 1 LARGE SMOOTHIE / **PREP TIME:** 5 MINUTES

GLUTEN-FREE, VEGAN

Chlorella powder is optional in this recipe, but it is a highly beneficial food. It is a freshwater alga that accelerates the body's natural detoxification process. Chlorella is also useful in binding to heavy metals and other toxins to remove them from the body. It contains protein, vitamin B_{12}, and iron, all of which are particularly important nutrients for vegetarians and vegans.

1 to 2 cups spinach

1 cup unsweetened original almond milk

1 teaspoon ground flaxseed

1 teaspoon shelled hemp seeds

½ frozen banana (optional)

¼ cup frozen avocado chunks (optional)

¼ cup vegan vanilla protein powder (optional)

1 teaspoon chlorella powder (optional)

3 ice cubes

In a blender, purée the spinach, almond milk, flaxseed, hemp seeds, banana (if using), avocado (if using), protein powder (if using), chlorella powder (if using), and ice. Drink immediately.

VARIATION TIP: The avocado is included to add a creamy texture and healthy fats, but you can omit it if you prefer. Feel free to add more greens, such as fresh mint, green apple, kale, cucumber, or parsley.

PER SERVING Calories: 180; Saturated Fat: 1g; Total Fat: 12g; Protein: 8g; Total Carbs: 7g; Fiber: 6g; Sodium: 407mg

Green Matcha Smoothie

MAKES: 1 LARGE SMOOTHIE / **PREP TIME:** 5 MINUTES

GLUTEN-FREE, VEGAN

Matcha is a clean energy source. Matcha is rich in antioxidants, boosts metabolism, and aids in the body's detoxification. The ingredients in this smoothie are strategically chosen to help your body function optimally.

1 cup spinach or kale

1 cup unsweetened original almond milk

½ green apple, peeled, cored, and chopped

¼ cup frozen avocado chunks (optional)

¼ cup vegan vanilla protein powder

1 teaspoon green matcha powder

1 teaspoon pure vanilla extract

In a blender, purée the spinach, almond milk, apple, avocado (if using), protein powder, matcha powder, and vanilla. Drink immediately.

PER SERVING Calories: 203; Saturated Fat: 0g; Total Fat: 4g; Protein: 23g; Total Carbs: 18g; Fiber: 5g; Sodium: 386mg

Immune-Boosting Smoothie

MAKES: 1 LARGE SMOOTHIE / PREP TIME: 5 MINUTES

GLUTEN-FREE, VEGAN

Among the best immunity boosters are citrus (grapefruit, lemons, limes, oranges), berries, veggies (especially red peppers), garlic, ginger, turmeric, and wheatgrass.

½ grapefruit, peeled and cubed

1 carrot, shredded

1 to 2 inches fresh ginger, minced

½ teaspoon ground turmeric

¼ cup vegan vanilla protein powder

1 cup unsweetened original almond milk

1. In a food processor, blend the grapefruit, carrots, ginger, and turmeric until smooth.
2. Add the protein powder and almond milk and blend again until smooth. Drink immediately.

VARIATION TIP: If you want to add a little natural sweetness, add half a frozen banana.

PER SERVING Calories: 203; Saturated Fat: 0g; Total Fat: 5g; Protein: 26g; Total Carbs: 15g; Fiber: 4g; Sodium: 473mg

Chocolate Dream Smoothie

MAKES: 1 LARGE SMOOTHIE / PREP TIME: 5 MINUTES

GLUTEN-FREE, VEGAN

This sweet-tasting smoothie provides plenty of nutrients and no empty calories.

1 cup unsweetened original almond milk

1 tablespoon almond butter

1 tablespoon cacao powder

1 tablespoon shelled hemp seeds

¼ cup vegan chocolate protein powder

3 to 4 ice cubes (add more to make it thicker, like ice cream)

½ frozen banana (optional)

In a blender, purée the almond milk, almond butter, cacao powder, hemp seeds, protein powder, ice cubes, and banana (if using). Drink immediately.

SUBSTITUTION TIP: You can use canned coconut milk instead of almond milk to make it creamier—just make sure it's unsweetened.

PER SERVING Calories: 385; Saturated Fat: 5g; Total Fat: 24g; Protein: 37g; Total Carbs: 17g; Fiber: 10g; Sodium: 463mg

Blueberry Bliss Smoothie

MAKES: 1 LARGE SMOOTHIE / PREP TIME: 5 MINUTES

GLUTEN-FREE, VEGAN

Blueberries and other dark berries like blackberries, raspberries, and cran-berries are high in antioxidants, fiber, and vitamins A and C. Antioxidants protect the body from free radicals, which can damage cells and lead to other health problems or harmful diseases. Free radicals are substances naturally created by the body when we breathe and digest food. The best way to reduce the risk of free radical damage is to consume foods that contain antioxidants, which is why it's important to add a lot of fruits and vegetables to your diet.

1 cup unsweetened vanilla almond milk

½ cup frozen blueberries

½ frozen banana

¼ cup vegan vanilla protein powder

1 tablespoon ground flaxseed

1 teaspoon pure vanilla extract

In a blender, purée the almond milk, blueberries, banana, protein powder, flaxseed, and vanilla. Drink immediately.

SUBSTITUTION TIP: Replace the banana with ½ cup of frozen blackberries to up the antioxidants even more.

VARIATION TIP: Make this a smoothie bowl by adding ice or more frozen fruit to thicken, and top with your favorite superfoods from your pantry.

PER SERVING Calories: 316; Saturated Fat: 1g; Total Fat: 9g; Protein: 29g; Total Carbs: 31g; Fiber: 8g; Sodium: 432mg

Pumpkin-Spiced Muffins

MAKES: 12 SERVINGS / **PREP TIME:** 10 MINUTES / **COOK TIME:** 15 MINUTES, PLUS 5 MINUTES TO COOL

GLUTEN-FREE, NUT-FREE, VEGETARIAN

If you do not have time to cook a pumpkin, canned pumpkin purée will work for this recipe—but avoid the added sugar of canned pumpkin pie filling.

1 teaspoon pure vanilla extract

¼ cup unsweetened applesauce or Apple Butter (page 86)

½ cup pumpkin purée (not pumpkin pie filling)

1 egg

1½ cups gluten-free rolled oats

½ cup vegan vanilla protein powder

¼ cup unsweetened coconut flakes

1 tablespoon ground flaxseed

2 teaspoons baking powder

1 teaspoon pumpkin pie spice

½ teaspoon ground cinnamon

¼ cup pumpkin seeds, for topping

1. Preheat the oven to 375°F. Line a muffin tin with liners.
2. In a medium bowl, combine the vanilla, applesauce, pumpkin purée, and egg.
3. In a large bowl, combine the oats, protein powder, coconut flakes, flaxseed, baking powder, pumpkin pie spice, and cinnamon.
4. Pour the wet ingredients into the dry ingredients and stir until incorporated.
5. Fill the muffin cups halfway, and top each with the pumpkin seeds.
6. Bake for 12 to 15 minutes, until cooked through and slightly golden.
7. Allow the muffins to cool for 5 minutes before serving.

BAKING TIP: When baking muffins, I like to keep a pan of water on the bottom shelf of the oven to keep the muffins moist.

SUBSTITUTION TIP: To make these muffins vegan, replace the egg with a mixture of 3 tablespoons of flaxseed and ⅓ cup of water.

PER SERVING Calories: 118; Saturated Fat: 3g; Total Fat: 6g; Protein: 7g; Total Carbs: 11g; Fiber: 3g; Sodium: 45mg

Super Seed Crackers

MAKES: 6 SERVINGS / **PREP TIME:** 20 MINUTES / **COOK TIME:** 55 MINUTES

GLUTEN-FREE, NUT-FREE, VEGAN

Every seed in these crackers provides the body with essential nutrients. Pumpkin seeds are a rich source of iron, sesame seeds are an excellent source of calcium, and flax, hemp, and chia seeds are all great sources of protein, fiber, and healthy omega-3 fatty acids. This combination will keep you fuller longer, which can prevent overeating. The chia seeds absorb liquid easily and work to bind the crackers.

1 cup water

½ cup chia seeds

½ cup pumpkin seeds

¼ cup ground flaxseed

¼ cup shelled hemp seeds

¼ cup sesame seeds

¼ cup sunflower seeds

2 garlic cloves, finely minced

¼ teaspoon salt (or favorite seasonings)

1. Preheat the oven to 375°F. Line a baking sheet with parchment paper.
2. In a large bowl, mix the water, chia seeds, pumpkin seeds, flaxseed, hemp seeds, sesame seeds, sunflower seeds, and garlic. Once well mixed, let sit for 10 minutes.
3. Stir the mixture again; the water should be absorbed by the seeds. Place the mixture on the prepared baking sheet and evenly spread with a spatula to cover the entire sheet.
4. Bake for 35 minutes. Flip the sheet of crackers (use two spatulas, if easier) and bake for 20 more minutes, until the seeds are golden.
5. Let cool and cut into squares to serve.

STORAGE TIP: Store leftovers in an airtight container. The crackers will stay fresh for up to one week, or will keep in the freezer for up to one month. Reheat in the oven to crisp up the crackers.

PER SERVING Calories: 232; Saturated Fat: 2g; Total Fat: 17g; Protein: 9g; Total Carbs: 13g; Fiber: 10g; Sodium: 101mg

Roasted Veggie Mix

MAKES: 4-6 SERVINGS / **PREP TIME:** 10 MINUTES / **COOK TIME:** 30 MINUTES

GLUTEN-FREE, NUT-FREE, VEGAN

Cruciferous vegetables (arugula, broccoli, Brussels sprouts, cabbage, cauliflower, and kale) are detox superstars. They are nutrient dense and low in calories, so you can fuel your cells and improve your body's detoxification process while losing weight. This recipe works great as a snack or a side. Change it up by topping the veggies with Lemon Tahini Dressing (page 75) or Roasted Red Pepper Dressing (page 74).

2 cups broccoli florets

2 cups cauliflower florets

2 tablespoons balsamic vinegar, divided

2 tablespoons avocado oil, divided

1 teaspoon salt, divided

2 cups green cabbage, shredded

2 cups red cabbage, shredded

1. Preheat the oven to 350°F.
2. Place the broccoli and cauliflower on a baking sheet and drizzle with 1 tablespoon of balsamic vinegar and 1 tablespoon of avocado oil. Mix by hand to evenly coat the veggies, and sprinkle with ½ teaspoon of salt.
3. On a second baking sheet, drizzle the remaining 1 tablespoon of balsamic vinegar and the remaining 1 tablespoon of avocado oil over the cabbage. Mix by hand to evenly coat and sprinkle with the remaining ½ teaspoon of salt.
4. Bake for 15 minutes. Flip the veggies and bake for an additional 15 minutes, until the veggies are roasted to a golden color.

STORAGE TIP: This is a great side dish for any number of meals, so if you'd like to double the recipe to have on hand, this dish will keep in the refrigerator for up to five days.

PER SERVING Calories: 114; Saturated Fat: 1g; Total Fat: 7g; Protein: 3g; Total Carbs: 11g; Fiber: 5g; Sodium: 528mg

Chipotle Barbecue Roasted Chickpeas

MAKES: 4 SERVINGS / **PREP TIME:** 5 MINUTES /
COOK TIME: 35 MINUTES

GLUTEN-FREE, NUT-FREE, VEGAN

Chickpeas make a great snack, salad topper, and vegan protein source for bowls and other dishes. If you do not like heat, substitute avocado oil for the hot sauce and regular chili powder for the ground chipotle chile.

1 (15.5-ounce) can chickpeas, drained and rinsed

1 tablespoon Frank's RedHot Original sauce

½ tablespoon avocado oil

1 teaspoon ground chipotle chile

1 teaspoon paprika

1 teaspoon dried oregano

1 teaspoon ground coriander

1 teaspoon garlic powder

1 teaspoon salt

½ teaspoon onion powder

1. Preheat the oven to 375°F and line a baking sheet with parchment paper.
2. Place the chickpeas in a large bowl. Pat them dry with a paper towel.
3. Add the hot sauce, avocado oil, chipotle chile, paprika, oregano, coriander, garlic powder, salt, and onion powder, and stir until evenly coated.
4. Carefully transfer the chickpeas to the baking sheet and bake for 20 minutes. Stir and bake for another 10 to 15 minutes, until the chickpeas are golden (longer, if you like them crunchier).
5. Remove and let sit for 5 minutes before eating.

PER SERVING Calories: 122; Saturated Fat: 0g; Total Fat: 4g; Protein: 6g; Total Carbs: 18g; Fiber: 5g; Sodium: 600mg

Homemade Trail Mix

MAKES: 4–8 SERVINGS / **PREP TIME:** 10 MINUTES / **COOK TIME:** 30 MINUTES

GLUTEN-FREE, VEGAN

This recipe can be made sweet or savory. Create a Cajun trail mix blend by replacing the almond butter, cinnamon, ginger, and pumpkin pie spice with hot sauce and Cajun spice blend. When your 10-day detox is completed, add ¼ cup of dried cranberries to this recipe for a boost of antioxidants.

¼ cup pecans

¼ cup almonds

¼ cup cashews

¼ cup sunflower seeds

¼ cup pumpkin seeds

¼ cup unsweetened large coconut flakes

1 tablespoon almond butter

½ tablespoon coconut oil

1 teaspoon ground cinnamon

¼ teaspoon ground ginger

½ teaspoon pumpkin pie spice

1. Preheat the oven to 375°F and line a baking sheet with parchment paper.
2. In a large bowl, combine the pecans, almonds, cashews, sunflower seeds, and pumpkin seeds. Add the coconut flakes, almond butter, coconut oil, cinnamon, ginger, and pumpkin pie spice and mix until the nuts and seeds are evenly coated.
3. Pour the mixture onto the baking sheet and bake for 25 to 30 minutes, until the nuts become fragrant and golden.
4. Remove and let cool. Place in an airtight container or portion into individual snack containers for an easy grab-and-go snack.

PER SERVING (calulations based on 4 servings)
Calories: 315; Saturated Fat: 9g; Total Fat: 28g; Protein: 8g; Total Carbs: 11g; Fiber: 5g; Sodium: 15mg

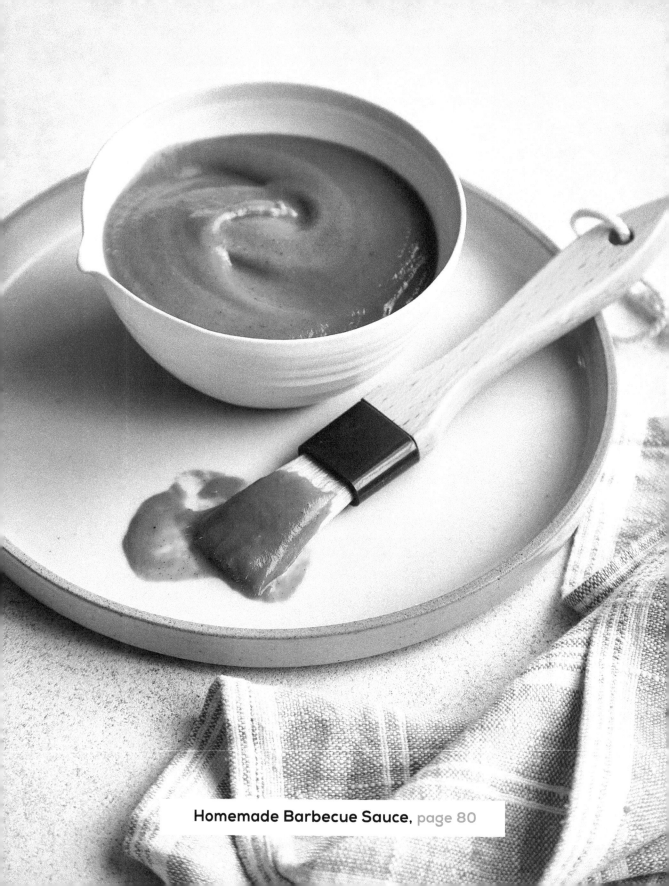

Homemade Barbecue Sauce, page 80

6

Condiments, Dips, and Sauces

One of the easiest ways to change up a dish is to try a different dressing or sauce. Instead of balsamic vinegar, try Roasted Red Pepper Dressing (page 74) or Ginger Lemon Dressing (page 76). The Cashew Cheese Sauce (page 84) can be used as a dip or added to any egg, meat, or veggie dish. The nutritional yeast in this dip is loaded with B vitamins—especially B_{12}—which is especially important for vegetarians and vegans. The Vegan Sour Cream (page 85) can punch up any Mexican dish, soup, or stew and tastes even better than store-bought sour cream.

Condiments and sauces tend to contain a lot of added sugar. Homemade Marinara Sauce (page 82) and Homemade Barbecue Sauce (page 80) are delicious low-sugar options. The Apple Butter (page 86) can be prepped on the weekend and used to replace honey, maple syrup, or sweeteners. The Cashew Fruit Dip (page 79) can top protein pancakes instead of maple syrup or replace dairy-filled fruit dips.

Roasted Red Pepper Dressing

MAKES: 1 CUP / **PREP TIME:** 10 MINUTES, PLUS OVERNIGHT TO SOAK

GLUTEN-FREE, VEGAN

This recipe can be made with jarred roasted red peppers, but if you prefer your peppers with a bit of a char, consider roasting them yourself.

½ cup cashews, soaked overnight and drained

2 to 3 large roasted red bell peppers, or 1 (12-ounce) jar roasted red peppers, drained

¼ cup olive oil

3 tablespoons balsamic vinegar

2 garlic cloves

1 teaspoon onion powder

1 teaspoon paprika

Pinch salt

Pinch freshly ground black pepper

In a blender, blend the cashews, peppers, olive oil, balsamic vinegar, garlic, onion powder, paprika, salt, and pepper until smooth.

STORAGE TIP: Stored in a jar, this dressing will keep in the refrigerator for up to one week.

TIME-SAVING TIP: If you don't have time to soak the cashews overnight, soak them in boiling water for 30 minutes.

PER SERVING (2 tablespoons) Calories: 81; Saturated Fat: 1g; Total Fat: 7g; Protein: 2g; Total Carbs: 5g; Fiber: 0g; Sodium: 16mg

Lemon Tahini Dressing

MAKES: ABOUT 1½ CUPS / **PREP TIME:** 10 MINUTES

GLUTEN-FREE, NUT-FREE, VEGAN

Tahini is simply sesame seeds that have been ground into a seed butter. This tasty spread is a great way to add antioxidants, iron, calcium, protein, and healthy fats to your meal. Sesame seeds also contain cholesterol-lowering phytosterols.

½ cup tahini

⅓ cup lemon juice

⅓ cup water

2 garlic cloves, peeled

¼ cup nutritional yeast

1 tablespoon toasted sesame oil

Pinch salt

Pinch freshly ground black pepper

In a food processor, blend the tahini, lemon juice, water, garlic, yeast, sesame oil, salt, and pepper until smooth. Additional water may be required; add 1 tablespoon at a time to achieve the desired consistency.

INGREDIENT TIP: Tahini is high in calories, so it should be used in moderation.

STORAGE TIP: Stored in a jar, this dressing can be kept in the refrigerator for up to one week.

PER SERVING (2 tablespoons) Calories: 85; Saturated Fat: 1g; Total Fat: 7g; Protein: 4g; Total Carbs: 4g; Fiber: 2g; Sodium: 26mg

Ginger Lemon Dressing

MAKES: ABOUT ¾ CUP / **PREP TIME:** 10 MINUTES

GLUTEN-FREE, NUT-FREE, VEGAN

Ginger adds a spicy kick to any recipe. It has many health benefits such as helping manage blood sugar levels and aiding in weight loss. Ginger can speed up metabolism and keep you feeling fuller longer.

½ cup freshly squeezed lemon juice

¼ cup olive oil

1 inch fresh ginger, minced

1 tablespoon Apple Butter (page 86)

Pinch sea salt or garlic salt

In a food processor, blend the lemon juice, olive oil, ginger, apple butter, and sea salt until smooth.

STORAGE TIP: Stored in a jar, this dressing will keep in the refrigerator for up to one week.

SUBSTITUTION TIP: If you do not have apple butter, substitute half a green apple or, if you are off the sugar detox, 1 tablespoon of maple syrup or raw coconut sugar.

PER SERVING (2 tablespoons) Calories: 84; Saturated Fat: 1g; Total Fat: 9g; Protein: 0g; Total Carbs: 2g; Fiber: 0g; Sodium: 5mg

Greek Dressing

MAKES: ABOUT 1 CUP / **PREP TIME:** 10 MINUTES, PLUS OVERNIGHT TO SOAK

GLUTEN-FREE, VEGAN

For this recipe, use store-bought Greek seasoning (read the ingredients list to be sure there's no added sugar) or make your own by combining the spices below in a small glass jar.

½ cup cashews, soaked overnight and drained

½ cup olive oil

3 tablespoons freshly squeezed lemon juice

2 tablespoons red wine vinegar

2 garlic cloves

1 tablespoon Greek seasoning (or 1 teaspoon dried oregano, 1 teaspoon dried basil, 1 teaspoon dried parsley, ½ teaspoon dried dill, and ½ teaspoon dried thyme)

Pinch salt

Pinch freshly ground black pepper

In a food processor, blend the cashews, olive oil, lemon juice, red wine, vinegar, garlic, Greek seasoning, salt, and pepper until smooth.

STORAGE TIP: Stored in a jar, this recipe will keep in the refrigerator for up to one week.

TIME-SAVING TIP: If you don't have time to soak the cashews overnight, soak them in boiling water for 30 minutes.

PER SERVING (2 tablespoons) Calories: 104; Saturated Fat: 2g; Total Fat: 11g; Protein: 1g; Total Carbs: 2g; Fiber: 0g; Sodium: 13mg

Balsamic Dressing

MAKES: ABOUT 1 CUP / **PREP TIME:** 10 MINUTES

GLUTEN-FREE, NUT-FREE, VEGAN

Sesame oil is made from sesame seeds and is used as a flavor enhancer in many Asian dishes. It has a nutty taste and aroma and is added to this balsamic dressing recipe to add flavor without sugar.

½ cup balsamic vinegar

½ cup olive oil

2 garlic cloves

1 scallion

1 tablespoon toasted sesame oil

Pinch salt

Pinch freshly ground black pepper

In a food processor, blend the balsamic vinegar, olive oil, garlic, scallion, sesame oil, salt, and pepper until smooth and the scallion is well minced.

STORAGE TIP: Stored in a jar, this dressing will keep in the refrigerator for up to one week.

VARIATION TIP: If you want to add a little sweetness to this dressing, you can add 1 tablespoon of Apple Butter (page 86).

PER SERVING (2 tablespoons) Calories: 139; Saturated Fat: 2g; Total Fat: 14g; Protein: 0g; Total Carbs: 3g; Fiber: 0g; Sodium: 23mg

Cashew Fruit Dip

MAKES: ABOUT 1¾ CUPS / **PREP TIME:** 10 MINUTES,
PLUS OVERNIGHT TO SOAK

GLUTEN-FREE, VEGAN

This recipe can be used as a fruit dip, a layer in chia pudding, or a topping for Coconut Chia Porridge (page 49) or Blueberry Protein Pancakes (page 55).

1 cup cashews, soaked overnight and drained

½ cup water

1 tablespoon lemon juice

½ cup fresh or frozen blueberries or strawberries

In a food processor, blend the cashews, water, lemon juice, and blueberries until smooth.

STORAGE TIP: Stored in a jar, this dip can be kept in the refrigerator for up to one week.

TIME-SAVING TIP: If you don't have time to soak the cashews overnight, soak them in boiling water for 30 minutes.

PER SERVING (¼ cup) Calories: 181; Saturated Fat: 2g; Total Fat: 13g; Protein: 5g; Total Carbs: 12g; Fiber: 2g; Sodium: 5mg

Homemade Barbecue Sauce

MAKES: 4-5 SERVINGS / PREP TIME: 10 MINUTES / COOK TIME: 50 MINUTES

GLUTEN-FREE, NUT-FREE, VEGAN

Caramelized onions are the secret to this sauce. You can caramelize any onion, but I find yellow onions work best. No Apple Butter (page 86) on hand? Use a large green apple, cored and puréed.

2 tablespoons avocado oil, divided

3 yellow onions, sliced

Pinch salt

3 garlic cloves, minced

1 tablespoon chili powder

½ teaspoon onion powder

½ teaspoon paprika

1 (6-ounce) can tomato paste

¼ cup Apple Butter (page 86)

¼ cup apple cider vinegar

1. In a large skillet over medium heat, add 1 tablespoon of avocado oil. Once the oil is heated, add the onions and salt.

2. Cook the onions for about 40 minutes, stirring every 5 minutes and scraping the fond (see Cooking Tip) that forms on the bottom of the pan. If it sticks too much to the bottom, deglaze by adding a little bit of water and scraping with a spoon. The onions are done when they are golden and start to smell like caramel. Deglaze the pan with 1 to 2 tablespoons water.

3. In a medium pot, add the remaining 1 tablespoon of avocado oil, garlic, chili powder, onion powder, and paprika and cook over medium heat for 1 to 2 minutes, until fragrant. Add the tomato paste, apple butter, and apple cider vinegar and reduce to low heat.

4. Transfer the onions to a blender or food processor and purée.
5. Add the puréed onions to the sauce mixture and cook for at least 10 minutes; the longer it cooks, the more flavor will develop.

COOKING TIP: As onions cook, they release water and steam, and some of their natural sugars accumulate on the bottom of the skillet. It might look like the onions are burning, but they are not; this sticky glaze is called the fond. Don't waste this flavorful substance on the bottom of the pan; it will dissolve and reabsorb quickly with a little liquid, so add a dash of broth, water, wine, or vinegar, and scrape it off the pan and back into the onions.

PER SERVING Calories: 189; Saturated Fat: 1g; Total Fat: 8g; Protein: 3g; Total Carbs: 29g; Fiber: 5g; Sodium: 68mg

Homemade Marinara Sauce

MAKES: 3–4 CUPS / **PREP TIME:** 5 MINUTES / **COOK TIME:** 30 MINUTES

GLUTEN-FREE, NUT-FREE, VEGAN

Making your own marinara sauce couldn't be easier. This recipe is customizable. Add caramelized onions to enhance the flavor or diced mushrooms and puréed spinach to increase the nutrient content.

1 (28-ounce) can diced tomatoes

½ red bell pepper

¼ cup fresh basil or 1 teaspoon dried basil

3 garlic cloves

½ yellow onion

⅓ cup olive oil

1 teaspoon dried oregano

1 teaspoon dried parsley

½ teaspoon salt

1. In a food processor, blend the tomatoes with their juices, red pepper, basil, garlic, and onion until smooth.
2. Pour the tomato mixture into a large pot and add the olive oil, oregano, parsley, and salt.
3. Simmer on medium-low heat for 30 minutes.

SUBSTITUTION TIP: You can use fresh tomatoes instead of canned diced tomatoes. Peel and dice 10 to 12 whole tomatoes (I like tomatoes on the vine as they have a sweet, juicy flavor), purée, and cook the same way. If I ever have tomatoes I'd like to use up, I make a sauce and toss them in.

PER SERVING (1 cup) Calories: 260; Saturated Fat: 3g; Total Fat: 23g; Protein: 3g; Total Carbs: 15g; Fiber: 4g; Sodium: 403mg

Peanut Curry Sauce

MAKES: 4–5 SERVINGS / **PREP TIME:** 10 MINUTES

GLUTEN-FREE, VEGAN

A good peanut sauce is neither too thick nor too runny. If the sauce seems too thick, add a little water or some fresh lime juice. If it's too runny, add more peanut butter. Peanut sauce adds a lot of flavor as well as healthy fat and protein. Although this sauce is nutrient dense, it is not low in calories, so enjoy it in moderation or pair it with low-calorie foods.

1 tablespoon avocado oil

2 garlic cloves

2 teaspoons grated fresh ginger

¾ cup water

⅓ cup natural peanut butter

3 tablespoons rice vinegar

2 tablespoons tamari

1 tablespoon Apple Butter (page 86)

1½ teaspoons yellow curry powder

In a food processor, blend the avocado oil, garlic, ginger, water, peanut butter, rice vinegar, tamari, apple butter, and yellow curry powder until smooth.

STORAGE TIP: Stored in a jar, this recipe will keep in the refrigerator for up to one week. If you do not use it all in a week, freeze it in a freezer-safe jar.

VARIATION TIP: If you are not a fan of curry, this recipe works great without it. After the 10-day detox, if you do not have apple butter prepared, you can substitute 1 tablespoon or coconut sugar or 1 tablespoon or pure maple syrup.

PER SERVING Calories: 192; Saturated Fat: 2g; Total Fat: 14g; Protein: 8g; Total Carbs: 8g; Fiber: 2g; Sodium: 508mg

Cashew Cheese Sauce

MAKES: 4–5 SERVINGS / **PREP TIME:** 10 MINUTES, PLUS OVERNIGHT TO SOAK

GLUTEN-FREE, VEGAN

This creamy cashew cheese sauce can be added to eggs, bowls, cauliflower rice, cut-up raw veggies, or anything that needs a little dairy-free cheese flavor.

1 cup cashews, soaked overnight and drained

½ cup unsweetened original almond milk

½ cup nutritional yeast

2 garlic cloves

½ teaspoon onion powder

¼ teaspoon salt

¼ teaspoon freshly ground black pepper

In a food processor, blend the cashews, almond milk, nutritional yeast, garlic, onion powder, salt, and pepper until smooth.

VARIATION TIP: You can sneak one or two cooked sweet potatoes and one or two cooked carrots into this cheese sauce to add more vegetables and create a thicker sauce; this is especially good if you have kids who are picky eaters and you're trying to get them to eat more veggies.

STORAGE TIP: Stored in a jar, this sauce will keep in the refrigerator for up to one week.

TIME-SAVING TIP: If you don't have time to soak the cashews overnight, soak them in boiling water for 30 minutes.

PER SERVING Calories: 210; Saturated Fat: 2g; Total Fat: 14g; Protein: 9g; Total Carbs: 13g; Fiber: 3g; Sodium: 176mg

Vegan Sour Cream

MAKES: ABOUT 1 CUP / **PREP TIME:** 10 MINUTES, PLUS OVERNIGHT TO SOAK

GLUTEN-FREE, VEGAN

This recipe is a highly satisfying alternative to traditional dairy sour cream, which can increase inflammation and cause blood sugar imbalances.

1 cup cashews, soaked overnight and drained

½ cup water

1 tablespoon apple cider vinegar

1 tablespoon lemon juice

1 tablespoon nutritional yeast

In a food processor, blend the cashews, water, apple cider vinegar, lemon juice, and nutritional yeast until smooth. Serve and enjoy.

COOKING TIP: If the sour cream is too thick, slowly add more water until the desired consistency is achieved.

STORAGE TIP: Stored in a glass jar, this sauce will keep in the refrigerator for up to one week.

TIME-SAVING TIP: If you don't have time to soak the cashews overnight, soak them in boiling water for 30 minutes.

PER SERVING (2 tablespoons) Calories: 61; Saturated Fat: 1g; Total Fat: 4g; Protein: 2g; Total Carbs: 3g; Fiber: 1g; Sodium: 2mg

Apple Butter

MAKES: ABOUT 4 CUPS / PREP TIME: 15 MINUTES / COOK TIME: 12 HOURS

GLUTEN-FREE, NUT-FREE, VEGAN

When a recipe needs a little sweetness, reach for this butter.

9 organic Granny Smith apples, peeled, cored, and diced

1 tablespoon ground cinnamon

1 tablespoon pure vanilla extract

1. In a slow cooker, combine the apples, cinnamon, and vanilla and mix to evenly coat.
2. Cover and cook on low for 12 hours, until the apples cook down and become golden.
3. Purée with an immersion blender until the mixture is smooth and thick; it will almost resemble a caramel sauce.

STORAGE TIP: Apple butter will keep for up to one week in an airtight jar in the refrigerator. If you don't think you will use all of it in that time, you can store the leftovers in ice cube trays in the freezer so you can easily add to a recipe as needed.

PER SERVING (2 tablespoons) Calories: 34; Saturated Fat: 0g; Total Fat: 0g; Protein: 0g; Total Carbs: 9g; Fiber: 2g; Sodium: 1mg

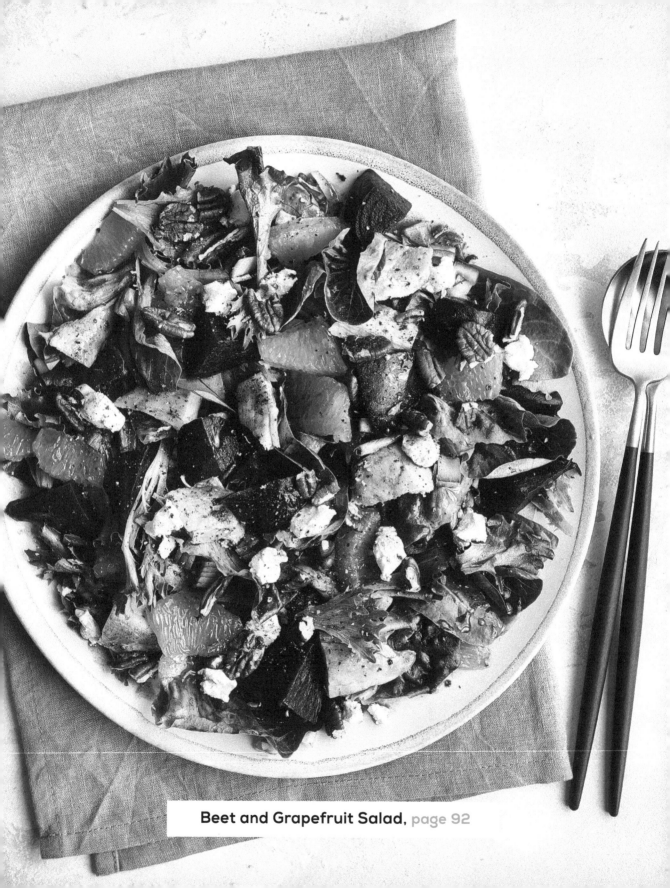

Beet and Grapefruit Salad, page 92

7

Salads and Soups

This chapter presents five salads loaded with nutrients and flavor.

Like the salads, this chapter's soups can be prepped and stored for future use. The Immune-Boosting Carrot Ginger Soup (page 99) is great when you feel run down. The Split Pea and Pumpkin Soup (page 97), packed with protein, iron, and zinc, is a perfect soup for vegans and vegetarians. The Black Bean Taco Stew (page 100) is a crowd-pleaser. Bring it to a potluck or serve it at your next dinner party.

Arugula and Quinoa Salad

MAKES: 2-3 SERVINGS / **PREP TIME:** 10 MINUTES

GLUTEN-FREE, NUT-FREE, VEGAN

Arugula is a member of the cruciferous vegetable family. It is loaded with vitamins (C, A, and K), beta carotene, and antioxidants. If you find arugula too peppery, mix it with baby spinach or kale.

1 cup cooled quinoa

1 to 2 cups arugula

½ red bell pepper, diced

1 cup chopped cucumber

1 beet, peeled and shredded

¼ cup chopped fresh cilantro (optional)

¼ cup pumpkin seeds

Balsamic Dressing (page 78)

1. In a large bowl, toss together the quinoa, arugula, red pepper, cucumber, beet, and cilantro (if using).
2. To serve, top with the pumpkin seeds and balsamic dressing.

PER SERVING Calories: 590; Saturated Fat: 4g; Total Fat: 27g; Protein: 18g; Total Carbs: 70g; Fiber: 9g; Sodium: 76mg

Apple and Almond Crunch Salad

MAKES: 2–3 SERVINGS / **PREP TIME:** 10 MINUTES

GLUTEN-FREE, VEGAN

After your 10-day detox is complete, I recommend adding ⅓ cup of dried cranberries to this recipe for more texture.

2 cups chopped arugula or spinach

1 cup finely chopped cauliflower

2 medium carrots, peeled and shredded (about 1 cup)

½ cup finely chopped red cabbage

½ cup chopped almonds

1 (15.5-ounce) can chickpeas, drained and rinsed

1 Granny Smith apple, cored and diced

Balsamic Dressing (page 78) or Ginger Lemon Dressing (page 76)

1. In a large bowl, toss together the arugula, cauliflower, carrots, cabbage, almonds, chickpeas, and apple.
2. Serve in individual portions and top with the dressing.

SUBSTITUTION TIP: You can substitute 1 to 2 cooked chicken breasts for the chickpeas.

PER SERVING Calories: 511; Saturated Fat: 1g; Total Fat: 17g; Protein: 22g; Total Carbs: 76g; Fiber: 22g; Sodium: 78mg

Beet and Grapefruit Salad

MAKES: 2–3 SERVINGS / PREP TIME: 10 MINUTES / COOK TIME: 50 MINUTES

GLUTEN-FREE

This recipe works with raw or cooked beets. An amazing root veggie loaded with vitamin C, fiber, folate, manganese, and potassium, beets are also rich in antioxidants and aid in liver detoxification.

2 beets, greens removed

2 tablespoons avocado oil, divided

2 boneless, skinless chicken breasts

Pinch salt

Pinch freshly ground black pepper

2 cups mixed greens

1 grapefruit, peeled and cubed

½ cup crushed pecans

¼ red onion, diced

2 tablespoons dairy-free goat cheese (optional)

Balsamic Dressing (page 78)

1. Preheat the oven to 400°F. Line a baking sheet with aluminum foil.
2. Coat the beets with 1 tablespoon of avocado oil and wrap in aluminum foil. Place them on one side of the baking sheet.
3. Place the chicken breasts on the other side of the baking sheet and coat with the remaining 1 tablespoon of avocado oil and season with salt and pepper.
4. Bake for 10 minutes, then flip the chicken and bake for an additional 15 minutes, until it is no longer pink in the center and has an internal temperature of 165°F. Transfer the chicken to a plate and let cool. Cut into bite-size cubes.
5. Meanwhile, bake the beets for an additional 25 minutes, for a total of 50 minutes. Remove the beets from the oven and allow them to cool. Remove the peels and cut into ½-inch cubes.

6. In a large bowl, combine the beets, chicken, mixed greens, grapefruit, pecans, red onion, and goat cheese (if using).
7. Top the salad with the dressing and serve.

VARIATION TIP: Make this recipe vegan by omitting the chicken and topping with your favorite vegan protein source.

PER SERVING Calories: 612; Saturated Fat: 6g; Total Fat: 42g; Protein: 39g; Total Carbs: 23g; Fiber: 7g; Sodium: 240mg

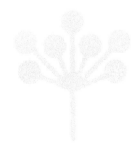

Mediterranean Chickpea Bowl

MAKES: 4-5 SERVINGS / **PREP TIME:** 10 MINUTES

GLUTEN-FREE, VEGAN

For extra flavor and crunch, you can roast the canned chickpeas: Simply toss them with olive oil and salt and pepper, spread them out on a rimmed baking sheet, and put them in a 375°F oven for 30 minutes. Stir them halfway through cooking.

2 cups arugula
or spring mix

1 (15.5-ounce) can
chickpeas, drained
and rinsed

20 Kalamata olives

1 cup cherry
tomatoes, diced

1 to 2 cups chopped
cucumber

½ cup diced red onion

1 cup cooked quinoa

Homemade Greek
dressing (page 77)

Dairy-free feta or goat
cheese (optional)

1. In individual bowls, layer equal amounts of the arugula, chickpeas, olives, tomatoes, cucumbers, onions, and quinoa.
2. To serve, top with the dressing and dairy-free feta cheese (if using).

PER SERVING Calories: 323; Saturated Fat: 3g; Total Fat: 17g; Protein: 12g; Total Carbs: 34g; Fiber: 8g; Sodium: 24mg

Salad Jars

When creating your jars, use any veggies you have on hand, aiming for a wide range of colors to ensure you are getting a variety of vitamins, minerals, and phytonutrients. Each jar should also contain a protein source; this recipe calls for quinoa, but you could use black beans, chickpeas, mung beans, lentils, tofu, hardboiled eggs, grilled chicken breast, cooked steak, salmon, shrimp, or pork chops.

1 cup cooked quinoa

1 large carrot, shredded

1 large beet, shredded

½ cup chopped red cabbage

½ cup chopped broccoli or cauliflower

½ cup chopped cucumber

½ cup halved cherry tomatoes

½ to 1 cup mixed greens

1 tablespoon shelled hemp seeds

Balsamic Dressing (page 78) or Ginger Lemon Dressing (page 76)

1. In 2 or 3 salad jars, layer equal parts of the quinoa, carrot, beet, cabbage, broccoli, cucumber, tomatoes, mixed greens, and hemp seeds.
2. To serve right away, top with your choice of dressing. To save for later, pack the dressing in a separate container and add in just before eating.

RECIPE TIP: If you need a little more for lunch, increase the amount of each ingredient and simply use a larger glass jar.

PER SERVING Calories: 219; Saturated Fat: 1g; Total Fat: 6g; Protein: 0g; Total Carbs: 32g; Fiber: 8g; Sodium: 587mg

Chicken Detox Stew

MAKES: 4-5 SERVINGS / PREP TIME: 20 MINUTES / COOK TIME: 30 MINUTES

GLUTEN-FREE, NUT-FREE

Turmeric is a spice superstar because it contains curcumin, a compound with anti-inflammatory benefits. To improve the bioavailability (absorption rate) of curcumin, consume turmeric with black pepper.

1 tablespoon avocado oil

2 boneless, skinless chicken breasts, cut into 1-inch cubes

3 garlic cloves, minced

¼ yellow onion, diced

2 cups chopped green cabbage

2 medium carrots, peeled and chopped

6 cups vegetable broth

1½ cups chopped broccoli

1 to 2 tablespoons yellow curry powder

1 teaspoon ground cumin

1 teaspoon ground turmeric

Pinch salt

Pinch freshly ground black pepper

Fresh cilantro, for garnish

1. In a large pot, heat the avocado oil over medium heat. Add the chicken, garlic, and onion and stir frequently, until the chicken is cooked through, 5 to 8 minutes.
2. Add the cabbage and carrots and stir for another 2 to 5 minutes.
3. Add the vegetable broth, broccoli, yellow curry powder, cumin, turmeric, salt, and pepper and cook for 20 minutes, until the vegetables are fork-tender.
4. Serve warm and garnish with fresh cilantro.

PER SERVING Calories: 300; Saturated Fat: 2g; Total Fat: 11g; Protein: 22g; Total Carbs: 28g; Fiber: 4g; Sodium: 546mg

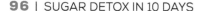

Split Pea and Pumpkin Soup

MAKES: 4–6 SERVINGS / PREP TIME: 10 MINUTES, PLUS OVERNIGHT TO SOAK / COOK TIME: 1 HOUR 30 MINUTES

GLUTEN-FREE, VEGAN

Split peas are an amazing source of plant-based protein. These legumes also contain iron and zinc, two nutrients to be mindful of when following a plant-based diet. Split peas are also high in soluble fiber, which helps bind and remove cholesterol-containing bile, reducing cholesterol levels. Split peas also help regulate blood sugar levels, providing a steady supply of energy due to their high fiber content.

2 cups dried yellow split peas

2 tablespoons avocado oil

½ onion, diced

2 garlic cloves, minced

6 cups vegetable broth

2 cups diced pumpkin or canned pumpkin purée (not pumpkin pie filling)

Salt

Freshly ground black pepper

Vegan Sour Cream (page 85), for garnish

Pumpkin seeds, for garnish

Ground nutmeg, for garnish

1. Rinse the split peas and soak them overnight in water. Drain and pat them dry.
2. In a large pot over medium to high heat, heat the avocado oil and sauté the onion and garlic.
3. Turn the heat down to medium and add the split peas, vegetable broth, pumpkin, and salt and pepper to taste.
4. Cover and simmer for 1½ hours, or until the peas are soft.
5. Top with a dollop of vegan sour cream, pumpkin seeds, and nutmeg.

PER SERVING Calories: 470; Saturated Fat: 1g; Total Fat: 9g; Protein: 26g; Total Carbs: 77g; Fiber: 29g; Sodium: 498mg

Indian-Spiced Turkey Stew

MAKES: 4-6 SERVINGS / **PREP TIME:** 15 MINUTES / **COOK TIME:** 30 MINUTES

GLUTEN-FREE, NUT-FREE

One of the best ways to boost the flavor in your meals without adding sugar is to experiment with spices. The spices in this stew add aroma and punch.

1 tablespoon avocado oil

½ yellow onion, diced

2 garlic cloves, minced

1 pound lean ground turkey

2 medium carrots, peeled and chopped

2 celery stalks, diced

½ head cauliflower, cut into florets

2 tablespoons yellow curry powder

1½ teaspoons ground cumin

1 teaspoon ground coriander

½ teaspoon garam masala

Pinch salt

Pinch freshly ground black pepper

6 cups vegetable broth

Fresh cilantro, for garnish

1. In a large pot, heat the avocado oil over medium heat. Add the onion, garlic, and turkey. Cook until the turkey is no longer pink, about 7 minutes.
2. Add the carrots, celery, and cauliflower and sauté for 2 to 3 minutes.
3. Add the yellow curry powder, cumin, coriander, garam masala, salt, and pepper and cook for another minute, until fragrant.
4. Pour in the broth and simmer on medium-low heat until the veggies are fork-tender, about 20 minutes.
5. Garnish with fresh cilantro before serving.

SUBSTITUTION TIP: Transform this stew into a vegan dish by substituting 2 cups of canned or cooked brown lentils for the turkey.

PER SERVING Calories: 236; Saturated Fat: 3g; Total Fat: 12g; Protein: 24g; Total Carbs: 9g; Fiber: 3g; Sodium: 128mg

Immune-Boosting Carrot Ginger Soup

MAKES: 4-6 SERVINGS / **PREP TIME:** 15 MINUTES / **COOK TIME:** 25 MINUTES

GLUTEN-FREE, NUT-FREE, VEGAN

Carrots contain vitamin A, which is crucial for cell production, growth, and development as well as for normal vision. Make this soup during the cold and flu season. Its ginger, garlic, and onion improve immune system function, and its red pepper provides vitamin C.

1 tablespoon
avocado oil

½ yellow onion

3 garlic cloves, minced

2 pounds carrots,
chopped

2 celery stalks,
chopped

1 to 2 tablespoons
minced fresh ginger

½ red bell
pepper, diced

4 cups vegetable broth

1½ (13.5-ounce)
cans coconut milk

Pinch salt

Pinch freshly ground
black pepper

Fresh cilantro,
for garnish

Pumpkin seeds, for
garnish (optional)

1. In a large pot, heat the avocado oil over medium heat. Add the onion, garlic, carrots, celery, and ginger and cook for 10 minutes, stirring occasionally.
2. Add the red pepper and cook for another 5 minutes.
3. Pour in the broth and simmer for 10 minutes, until the veggies are fork-tender.
4. Remove from the heat and add the coconut milk, reserving ¼ cup for garnish.
5. Using an immersion blender, purée the soup.
6. To serve, drizzle with the reserved coconut milk and season with salt and pepper. Garnish with cilantro and pumpkin seeds (if using).

COOKING TIP: If you do not own an immersion blender, use a blender or food processor.

PER SERVING Calories: 341; Saturated Fat: 16g; Total Fat: 22g; Protein: 5g; Total Carbs: 36g; Fiber: 7g; Sodium: 655mg

Black Bean Taco Stew

MAKES: 4-6 SERVINGS / PREP TIME: 10 MINUTES / COOK TIME: 40 MINUTES

GLUTEN-FREE

This stew's taco spice blend is healthier than prepackaged versions, which often contain a lot of sugar, salt, and wheat.

1 tablespoon avocado oil

½ yellow onion, diced

3 garlic cloves, minced

1 pound ground beef

2 tablespoons chili powder

1 tablespoon ground cumin

1 teaspoon onion powder

1 teaspoon garlic powder

1 teaspoon salt

½ teaspoon freshly ground black pepper

½ teaspoon dried oregano

1. In a large pot, heat the avocado oil over medium heat. Add the onion, garlic, and beef and cook until the beef is no longer pink, 6 to 8 minutes.

2. Add the chili powder, cumin, onion powder, garlic powder, salt, pepper, oregano, and paprika and cook for 1 minute, or until fragrant.

3. Add the tomatoes with their juices, soup mix, black beans, yellow pepper, orange pepper, and broth and simmer on low for a minimum of 30 minutes.

4. Garnish with your choice of toppings.

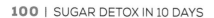

½ teaspoon paprika

1 (28-ounce) can diced tomatoes

1 (16-ounce) pouch multi-bean soup mix

1 (15-ounce) can black beans, drained and rinsed

½ yellow bell pepper, chopped

½ orange bell pepper, chopped

2 cups vegetable broth

Chopped lettuce, tomato, and avocado, for garnish (optional)

Vegan Sour Cream (page 85), for garnish (optional)

SUBSTITUTION TIP: Make this a vegan meal by omitting the ground beef.

PER SERVING Calories: 745; Saturated Fat: 4g; Total Fat: 14g; Protein: 59g; Total Carbs: 101g; Fiber: 28g; Sodium: 813mg

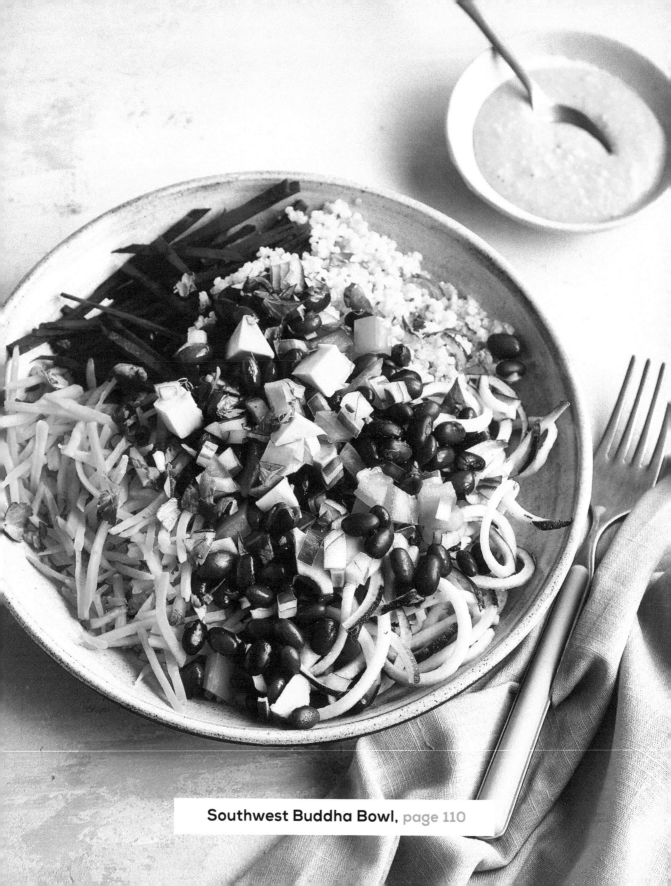

Southwest Buddha Bowl, page 110

8

Vegan and Vegetarian Mains

This chapter is filled with nutritionally sound recipes for vegans and vegetarians to ensure adequate protein, healthy fats and carbs, fiber, and veggies. The Lentil and Mushroom Burgers (page 114), Slow Cooker Barbecue Lentil Chili (page 131), Vegan Shepherd's Pie with Cauliflower Mash (page 130), and Zoodle Lasagna with Basil Cashew Cheese (page 132) are the perfect comfort foods to maintain healthy eating and achieve weight loss goals.

Bowls seem to be all the rage. Check out the Southwest Buddha Bowls (page 110), Portobello Fajita Bowls (page 128), Vegan Taco Bowls (page 127), Moroccan-Spiced Chickpea Bowls (page 126), and Black Bean Enchilada Bowls (page 124).

Thai-Inspired Red Curry with Cauliflower Rice

MAKES: 4-5 SERVINGS / **PREP TIME:** 10 MINUTES / **COOK TIME:** 25 MINUTES

GLUTEN-FREE, NUT-FREE, VEGAN

Thai food has many health benefits: Ginger is great for improving digestion and reducing inflammation, red peppers are an excellent source of vitamin C, chickpeas are a wonderful source of vegan protein and fiber, and coconut milk is a healthy fat that contains medium chain triglycerides (MCT), which help keep you satiated.

2 tablespoons avocado oil, divided

½ yellow onion, diced

1 inch fresh ginger, minced

2 garlic cloves, minced

1 red bell pepper, diced

1 yellow bell pepper, diced

3 tablespoons Thai red curry paste

1½ (13.5-ounce) cans coconut milk

2 (15.5-ounce) cans chickpeas, drained and rinsed

1. In a large skillet, heat 1 tablespoon of avocado oil over medium heat. Add the onion and sauté for 1 minute. Add the ginger and garlic and cook until fragrant, about 30 seconds, stirring frequently.

2. Add the red and yellow peppers and cook until fork-tender, about 5 minutes, then add the curry paste, coconut milk, chickpeas, tamari, rice vinegar, spinach, salt, and pepper. Simmer over low heat for 10 to 15 minutes.

3. Meanwhile, in a separate large skillet, heat the remaining 1 tablespoon of avocado oil over medium heat. Sauté the cauliflower rice for 5 minutes, until soft and translucent.

2 tablespoons tamari

½ tablespoon
rice vinegar

2 cups chopped baby
spinach or kale

Pinch salt

Pinch freshly ground
black pepper

2 cups cauliflower rice

Fresh cilantro,
for garnish

4. To serve, fill a third of a bowl with cauliflower rice and the rest with the creamy Thai curry mixture. Garnish with fresh cilantro.

STORAGE TIP: This dish is freezer friendly. Place leftovers in individual-portion containers and freeze for up to one month.

VARIATION TIP: To save a step when making this dish, buy frozen cauliflower rice; this also allows you to save time and cook the exact amount you need. If you have fresh cauliflower rice and made too much, you can freeze the leftovers.

PER SERVING Calories: 677; Saturated Fat: 29g; Total Fat: 42g; Protein: 21g; Total Carbs: 62g; Fiber: 15g; Sodium: 847mg

Slow Cooker Thai-Inspired Coconut Curry Chickpea Soup

MAKES: 4-5 SERVINGS / **PREP TIME:** 10 MINUTES / **COOK TIME:** 8 HOURS

GLUTEN-FREE, NUT-FREE, VEGAN

The lemongrass in this soup is optional, but it is highly recommended. A staple in Thai cooking, lemongrass is used more for its aroma than its flavor. It pairs well with dishes that contain coconut milk and Indian or Thai spices.

2 garlic cloves, minced

1 inch fresh ginger, minced

2 (15.5-ounce) cans chickpeas, drained and rinsed

4 cups vegetable broth

3 tablespoons red curry paste

1. In a slow cooker, combine the garlic, ginger, chickpeas, broth, red curry paste, coconut milk, red pepper, carrots, and lemongrass (if using).
2. Cover and cook on high for 4 hours or on low for 8 hours.
3. Add the spinach 5 to 10 minutes before serving.

COOKING TIP: If you do not have a slow cooker, cook this dish in a large pot on the stove. Add the garlic, ginger, red pepper, and carrots over medium heat and cook for 3 minutes. Add the chickpeas, broth, red curry paste, coconut milk, tamari, and lemongrass (if using). Cook for 20 minutes, or until the vegetables are fork-tender, then add the spinach in the last 5 minutes of cooking.

1½ (13.5-ounce) cans coconut milk

1 red bell pepper, diced

2 medium carrots, peeled and chopped

3 inches lemongrass (optional)

2 to 3 cups chopped spinach or kale

INGREDIENT TIP: If using lemongrass, chop off the ends and use the bottom 3 inches only. Peel off the tough outer layer and smash with a meat tenderizer or the bottom of a glass bottle to release the fragrant oils. Place the smashed lemongrass in the slow cooker and use as you would a bay leaf, removing before serving. You can save the top portion of the lemongrass to add to stock or to make lemongrass tea. If you are not going to use it right away, wrap it in foil and freeze for up to one month.

PER SERVING Calories: 534; Saturated Fat: 31g; Total Fat: 39g; Protein: 19g; Total Carbs: 66g; Fiber: 17g; Sodium: 738mg

Chickpeas with Cauliflower Rice

MAKES: 4-5 SERVINGS / PREP TIME: 10 MINUTES / COOK TIME: 25 MINUTES

GLUTEN-FREE, NUT-FREE, VEGAN

This recipe's chickpeas and coconut milk pack a protein punch. If you want more heat, add more chili powder, curry powder, and garam masala.

2 tablespoons avocado oil, divided

½ yellow onion, diced

2 garlic cloves, minced

1 inch fresh ginger, grated

1 tablespoon yellow curry powder

2 teaspoons chili powder

1 teaspoon garam masala

1 teaspoon ground cumin

½ teaspoon ground turmeric

½ teaspoon salt

1 (14.5-ounce) can diced tomatoes

1½ (13.5-ounce) cans coconut milk

2 (15.5-ounce) cans chickpeas, drained and rinsed

2 cups cauliflower rice

Fresh cilantro, for garnish

1. In a large skillet, heat 1 tablespoon of avocado oil over medium heat. Add the onion, garlic, and ginger and cook for 4 minutes. Add the yellow curry powder, chili powder, garam masala, cumin, turmeric, and salt and cook for 1 more minute, or until fragrant.
2. Add the tomatoes with their juices, coconut milk, and chickpeas and simmer over low heat for 15 to 20 minutes.
3. In a medium skillet, heat the remaining 1 tablespoon of avocado oil over medium heat. Add the cauliflower rice and cook for 5 minutes, until soft.
4. Serve the chickpeas over the cauliflower rice and garnish with cilantro.

COOKING TIP: To thicken the sauce, add 1 tablespoon of tapioca starch.

PER SERVING Calories: 648; Saturated Fat: 28g; Total Fat: 38g; Protein: 21g; Total Carbs: 63g; Fiber: 18g; Sodium: 549mg

Eggplant Parm

MAKES: 4-5 SERVINGS / PREP TIME: 20 MINUTES / COOK TIME: 40 MINUTES

GLUTEN-FREE, VEGAN

Because eggplants are low in protein, this dish calls for almond flour, hummus, and vegan Parmesan cheese.

1 to 2 cups almond flour

1 tablespoon Italian seasoning

¼ cup vegan Parmesan cheese, plus extra for topping (optional)

1 (8-ounce) container garlic hummus

3 to 4 table-spoons water

1 large eggplant, peeled and cut into ½-inch-thick pieces

1 batch Homemade Marinara Sauce (page 82)

2 to 4 zucchinis, spiralized into zoodles (3 to 4 cups)

1. Preheat the oven to 350°F. Line a baking sheet with parchment paper.
2. Fill a small bowl halfway with almond flour. Add the Italian seasoning and vegan Parmesan cheese (if using).
3. Put the hummus in another small bowl and add the water in a slow, steady stream, mixing until it has an egg-like consistency.
4. Dip the eggplant into the hummus wash, evenly coating. Dip in the almond flour mixture and place on the baking sheet.
5. Bake for 15 to 20 minutes, flip, and bake for an additional 15 to 20 minutes.
6. In a medium pot, heat the marinara sauce.
7. Just before serving, place the zoodles on an oven-safe plate and warm in the oven for about 3 minutes.
8. Pour the marinara sauce over the zoodles and top with the eggplant and additional vegan Parmesan cheese (if using).

RECIPE TIP: Handheld spiralizers can be purchased at most stores for $10 to $20. If you do not own a spiralizer, you can purchase spiralized zoodles in most grocery stores.

PER SERVING Calories: 508; Saturated Fat: 5g; Total Fat: 36g; Protein: 14g; Total Carbs: 40g; Fiber: 16g; Sodium: 603mg

Southwest Buddha Bowls

MAKES: 4 SERVINGS / **PREP TIME:** 15 MINUTES, PLUS OVERNIGHT TO SOAK

GLUTEN-FREE, VEGAN

This bowl works equally well with the Southwest dressing below and the Roasted Red Pepper Dressing (page 74).

FOR THE SOUTHWEST DRESSING

¼ cup freshly squeezed lime juice

½ tablespoon red wine vinegar

¼ cup olive oil

¼ cup cashews, soaked overnight and drained

2 garlic cloves, minced

½ teaspoon ground cumin

½ teaspoon salt

½ teaspoon garlic salt

½ teaspoon chili powder

½ tablespoon Frank's RedHot original sauce (optional)

FOR THE BUDDHA BOWLS

1 (15-ounce) can black beans, drained and rinsed

1 to 2 ripe avocados, cubed

2 tomatoes, diced

¼ cup red onion, chopped (optional)

2 to 4 zucchinis, spiralized into zoodles (3 to 4 cups)

1 cup cooked quinoa

1 carrot, shredded

1 beet, shredded

Lime juice, for garnish (optional)

Frank's RedHot Original sauce, for garnish (optional)

Fresh cilantro, for garnish (optional)

1 red bell pepper, chopped, for garnish (optional)

TO MAKE THE SOUTHWEST DRESSING

In a food processor, blend the lime juice, red wine vinegar, olive oil, cashews, garlic, cumin, salt, garlic salt, chili powder, and hot sauce (if using) until smooth.

TO MAKE THE BUDDHA BOWL

1. In a large bowl, mix the black beans, avocados, tomatoes, and onion (if using).
2. To serve, assemble individual bowls by equally distributing the zoodles, quinoa, carrots, and beet. Top with the black bean mixture.
3. Drizzle the Southwest dressing over the top and, if desired, garnish with lime juice, hot sauce, fresh cilantro, or red pepper.

SERVING TIP: If you're making this dish ahead of time and won't be consuming it within 24 hours, omit the avocado until just before serving.

TIME-SAVING TIP: If you don't have time to soak the cashews overnight, soak them in boiling water for 30 minutes.

PER SERVING Calories: 434; Saturated Fat: 3g; Total Fat: 24g; Protein: 13g; Total Carbs: 47g; Fiber: 14g; Sodium: 348mg

Peanut Chickpea Tacos in Lettuce Wraps

MAKES: 4-5 SERVINGS / **PREP TIME:** 15 MINUTES / **COOK TIME:** 10 MINUTES

GLUTEN-FREE, VEGAN

This recipe works really well with all-natural almond butter instead of peanut butter. No matter which nut butter you use, be sure to read the ingredients list to ensure that the only ingredient is nuts. Avoid butters with added sugar or salt.

FOR THE PEANUT SAUCE

1 tablespoon olive or avocado oil

2 garlic cloves, minced

2 teaspoons grated fresh ginger

¾ cup water, plus extra as needed

⅓ cup natural peanut butter

3 tablespoons rice vinegar

2 tablespoons tamari

½ tablespoon Apple Butter (page 86)

TO MAKE THE PEANUT SAUCE

In a small saucepan over medium heat, add the avocado oil, garlic, and ginger and sauté for 1 minute. Add the water, peanut butter, rice vinegar, tamari, and apple butter and cook for 5 minutes, until the sauce thickens.

TO MAKE THE TACOS

1. Heat the avocado oil in a large skillet over medium heat and add the garlic and onion. Cook for 4 minutes, then add the chickpeas.
2. Add the cabbage and carrots and cook for 1 to 2 minutes.
3. Add half of the peanut sauce and stir to coat the chickpeas. Cook for 1 minute and remove from the heat. If you like your tacos extra saucy, add more peanut sauce to your preference.

FOR THE TACOS

1 tablespoon
avocado oil

2 garlic cloves, minced

⅓ yellow onion, diced

1 (15.5-ounce) can
chickpeas, drained
and rinsed

1 cup finely chopped
red cabbage

2 medium carrots,
peeled and shredded

1 head romaine lettuce,
leaves separated

¼ cup chopped peanuts
or slivered almonds

Fresh cilantro,
for garnish

Lime juice, for garnish

4. Assemble the tacos by spooning equal
amounts of the chickpea mixture into
romaine lettuce leaves. Garnish with
chopped peanuts, fresh cilantro, and a little
lime juice.

PER SERVING Calories: 383; Saturated Fat: 4g;
Total Fat: 23g; Protein: 16g; Total Carbs: 31g; Fiber: 9g;
Sodium: 542mg

Lentil and Mushroom Burgers

MAKES: 6 SERVINGS / **PREP TIME:** 10 MINUTES / **COOK TIME:** 40 MINUTES

GLUTEN-FREE, VEGAN

These burgers contain four protein sources: quinoa, lentils, almond flour, and cremini mushrooms. Quinoa is considered a plant-based complete protein source because it contains all nine essential amino acids. Lentils are a wonderful source of iron, mushrooms are high in zinc, and nutritional yeast contains vitamin B_{12}.

1 tablespoon avocado oil

½ yellow onion, diced

3 garlic cloves, minced

1 (8-ounce) package cremini mushrooms, sliced

2 cups cooked brown lentils

3 tablespoons ground flaxseed

⅓ cup water

¾ cup cooked quinoa

1. Preheat the oven to 350°F and line a baking sheet with parchment paper.
2. In a large skillet, heat the avocado oil over medium heat and sauté the onion, garlic, and mushrooms for about 5 minutes, until the mushrooms are soft and dark brown.
3. Transfer the mixture to a food processor and pulse until well combined. Add the lentils and pulse again.
4. To create the vegan egg mixture, in a small bowl, combine the flaxseed and water and let sit for 5 to 10 minutes, until the mixture thickens to an egg-like consistency.
5. Pour the lentil mixture into a large bowl and stir in the quinoa, vegan egg mixture, nutritional yeast, and almond flour. Mix until well combined.

1 tablespoon nutritional yeast

½ to 1 cup almond flour or gluten-free bread crumbs

1 head iceberg lettuce, leaves separated

2 tomatoes, sliced, for garnish (optional)

Homemade Barbecue Sauce (page 80; optional)

6. Form the mixture into 6 patties, packing the edges well.
7. Place on the baking sheet and bake for 15 minutes. Flip and bake for an additional 15 minutes.
8. Place each burger patty between two leaves of lettuce and garnish with tomato slices and barbecue sauce, if desired.

STORAGE TIP: If you have leftover burgers, individually wrap them and freeze for up to one month.

PER SERVING Calories: 190; Saturated Fat: 1g; Total Fat: 6g; Protein: 11g; Total Carbs: 26g; Fiber: 8g; Sodium: 16mg

Mexican-Inspired Stuffed Peppers

MAKES: 4-6 SERVINGS / **PREP TIME**: 10 MINUTES / **COOK TIME**: 50 MINUTES

GLUTEN-FREE, NUT-FREE, VEGAN

Traditional stuffed peppers are often loaded with rice and corn, making them unsuitable for this detox. Enjoy this clean version with cauliflower rice, quinoa, black beans, and Mexican spices. For a yummy variation, try them topped with Cashew Cheese Sauce (page 84).

1 (28-ounce) can diced tomatoes

1 (15-ounce) can black beans, drained and rinsed

1 (4-ounce) can diced green chiles, drained (optional)

2 garlic cloves, minced

½ cup cooked quinoa

½ cup cauliflower rice

1 tablespoon chili powder

1 teaspoon ground cumin

1 teaspoon onion powder

Salt

Freshly ground black pepper

4 red bell peppers, cored and cut in half lengthwise

1. Preheat the oven to 350°F.
2. In a large bowl, combine about three-quarters of the diced tomatoes, the black beans, green chiles (if using), garlic, quinoa, cauliflower rice, chili powder, cumin, and onion powder, and season with salt and pepper to taste.
3. Coat the bottom of a large casserole dish with the remaining tomatoes. Lay the peppers on top of the tomatoes, open-side up.
4. Stuff the peppers with the black bean mixture, cover with foil, and bake for 40 minutes.
5. Remove the foil and cook for 10 more minutes, until the peppers are softened but not mushy.

COOKING TIP: The peppers can be stuffed and refrigerated one day ahead of time for a quick and easy weeknight dinner; simply bake for 50 minutes rather than 40 before removing the foil.

PER SERVING Calories: 206; Saturated Fat: 0g; Total Fat: 2g; Protein: 11g; Total Carbs: 41g; Fiber: 11g; Sodium: 40mg

Buffalo Chickpea Tacos in Lettuce Wraps

MAKES: 5–6 SERVINGS / **PREP TIME:** 10 MINUTES / **COOK TIME:** 10 MINUTES

GLUTEN-FREE, VEGAN

This recipe puts a spicy twist on chickpea tacos. If you don't like heat, replace the hot sauce with Homemade Barbecue Sauce (page 80).

1 tablespoon vegan butter or ghee

¼ to ⅓ cup Frank's RedHot Original sauce

1 tablespoon avocado oil

2 garlic cloves, minced

¼ yellow onion, diced

1 (15.5-ounce) can chickpeas, drained and rinsed

1 head romaine lettuce, leaves separated

Vegan Sour Cream (page 85; optional)

Tomatoes, diced, for garnish (optional)

Avocado, diced, for garnish (optional)

Fresh cilantro, for garnish (optional)

Red and/or orange bell pepper, diced, for garnish (optional)

1. In a small pot, melt the butter and stir in the hot sauce.
2. In a large skillet over medium heat, add the avocado oil, garlic, and onion and sauté for 3 minutes. Add the chickpeas and buffalo sauce and cook for 5 minutes. Remove from the heat.
3. Place the lettuce leaves on a plate. To serve, spoon equal amounts of the buffalo chickpea mixture onto the lettuce leaves. Garnish with your favorite toppings (if using).

PER SERVING Calories: 168; Saturated Fat: 6g; Total Fat: 9g; Protein: 7g; Total Carbs: 19g; Fiber: 5g; Sodium: 42mg

Greek Burgers

MAKES: 4–6 BURGERS / **PREP TIME:** 10 MINUTES / **COOK TIME:** 25 MINUTES

GLUTEN-FREE, VEGAN

Make a double batch of these burgers so you can individually wrap some of them and put them in the freezer. They're a great meatless option for barbecues or parties.

3 tablespoons ground flaxseed

⅓ cup water

1 (15-ounce) can black beans, drained and rinsed

¼ cup chopped fresh dill

2 large garlic cloves, minced

1 teaspoon onion powder

½ cup gluten-free rolled oats

⅓ cup gluten-free bread crumbs

1. Preheat the oven to 350°F. Line a baking sheet with parchment paper.
2. To make your vegan egg mixture, in a small bowl, combine the flaxseed and water and set aside for 5 to 10 minutes, until thickened.
3. In a large bowl, mash the black beans into a semi-paste. Stir in the dill, garlic, onion powder, oats, bread crumbs, olive oil, tamari, Greek seasoning, dairy-free feta cheese (if using), olives, red pepper, salt, and pepper. Add the flaxseed mixture last. Mix until well combined.
4. Shape the mixture into 4 to 6 patties and place on the baking sheet. Pack the patties tightly, especially around the edges to help hold them together during baking.

½ tablespoon extra-virgin olive oil

1 to 2 tablespoons tamari or coconut aminos

2 tablespoons Greek seasoning

¼ cup crumbled dairy-free feta cheese (optional)

10 black olives, pitted and sliced

1 roasted red bell pepper, finely diced

½ teaspoon salt

Pinch freshly ground black pepper

Homemade Greek Dressing (page 77)

Lettuce, for garnish

Tomato, sliced, for garnish

5. Bake the patties for 10 to 15 minutes. Gently flip them, then bake for 10 to 15 minutes more, until firm. Top with the Greek dressing, lettuce, and tomato.

INGREDIENT TIP: You can buy premade Greek seasoning from most grocery stores. If you can't find it or would prefer to make your own, you can do so by combining the dry ingredients from the recipe for Greek Dressing on page 77.

STORAGE TIP: These burgers freeze very well. If you have leftovers, wrap them individually and freeze for up to three months. Reheat in the oven for an easy lunch or dinner.

PER SERVING Calories: 208; Saturated Fat: 1g; Total Fat: 5g; Protein: 10g; Total Carbs: 34g; Fiber: 8g; Sodium: 913mg

Lasagna-Stuffed Portobello Mushrooms

MAKES: 4-6 SERVINGS / **PREP TIME:** 10 MINUTES, PLUS OVERNIGHT TO SOAK / **COOK TIME:** 20 MINUTES

GLUTEN-FREE, VEGAN

This lasagna gets its flavor from basil cashew cheese and marinara sauce.

FOR THE VEGAN BASIL CASHEW CHEESE SAUCE

1½ cups cashews soaked overnight and drained

½ to 1 cup unsweetened original almond milk

¼ cup fresh basil

1 teaspoon Italian seasoning

1 tablespoon nutritional yeast

2 garlic cloves

Pinch salt

Pinch freshly ground black pepper

FOR THE MUSHROOMS

4 to 6 portobello mushrooms, stems and gills removed

1 to 2 tablespoons olive oil

1 batch Homemade Marinara Sauce (page 82)

1½ cups chopped spinach

½ cup chopped fresh basil

TO MAKE THE VEGAN BASIL CASHEW CHEESE SAUCE

In a food processor, blend the cashews, almond milk, basil, Italian seasoning, nutritional yeast, garlic, salt, and pepper until smooth. If the mixture is not to your desired thickness, you can add more almond milk and pulse until well combined.

TO MAKE THE MUSHROOMS

1. Preheat the oven to 400°F.
2. Brush the mushrooms all over with olive oil.
3. Pour 2 cups of marinara into a large casserole dish and add the mushrooms gill-side up.
4. Spoon ¼ cup of marinara sauce into each mushroom.
5. Fill each mushroom with the cheese sauce, spinach, and basil.
6. Bake for 20 minutes, or until the mushrooms are soft and the cashew cheese crisps up.

TIME-SAVING TIP: If you don't have time to soak the cashews overnight, soak the cashews in boiling water for 30 minutes.

PER SERVING Calories: 613; Saturated Fat: 7g; Total Fat: 47g; Protein: 18g; Total Carbs: 36g; Fiber: 9g; Sodium: 463mg

Mushroom Stroganoff with Garlic Cauliflower Mash

MAKES: 5–6 SERVINGS / PREP TIME: 10 MINUTES, PLUS
OVERNIGHT TO SOAK / COOK TIME: 10 MINUTES

GLUTEN-FREE, VEGAN

Cashews are a great replacement for dairy-filled cream sauces. They're packed with protein and healthy fats. Cashews are also an excellent source of antioxidants, potassium, iron, magnesium, and vitamin B_6.

FOR THE CASHEW SAUCE

1½ cups cashews, soaked overnight and drained

2 cups unsweetened original almond milk, plus more as needed

½ teaspoon garlic salt

¼ cup nutritional yeast

TO MAKE THE CASHEW SAUCE

In a food processor, blend the cashews, almond milk, garlic salt, and nutritional yeast until liquefied.

TO MAKE THE STROGANOFF

1. In a large skillet, heat the avocado oil over medium heat. Add the mushrooms, garlic, and onion and sauté until the mushrooms are browned, about 5 minutes.
2. Pour the cashew sauce over the mushrooms and heat. If the mixture becomes too thick, thin by adding almond milk. Add salt and pepper to taste.

FOR THE STROGANOFF

1 tablespoon avocado oil

2 (8-ounce) packages sliced cremini mushrooms

3 garlic cloves, minced

¼ yellow onion, finely chopped

Salt

Freshly ground black pepper

FOR THE CAULIFLOWER MASH

1 tablespoon avocado oil

4 cups cauliflower rice

1 tablespoon nutritional yeast

TO MAKE THE CAULIFLOWER MASH

1. In another large skillet, heat the avocado oil over medium heat. Add the cauliflower rice and nutritional yeast. Cook for 5 minutes, until the rice is translucent and soft. If you prefer a smoother texture, blend with an immersion blender to make it more like mashed potatoes.

2. To serve, fill individual bowls halfway with cauliflower mash and the other half with the stroganoff.

COOKING TIP: If you do not have an immersion blender you can use a regular potato masher instead. If you prefer a thicker cashew sauce, add 1 tablespoon of tapioca starch.

PER SERVING Calories: 387; Saturated Fat: 3g; Total Fat: 24g; Protein: 19g; Total Carbs: 28g; Fiber: 8g; Sodium: 111mg

Black Bean Enchilada Bowls

MAKES: 4-6 SERVINGS / PREP TIME: 10 MINUTES / COOK TIME: 25 MINUTES

GLUTEN-FREE, VEGAN

Enchiladas can be high in calories and sugar because they are typically served in wraps with cheese and rice. This version eliminates the wraps and cheese and replaces the rice with zoodles.

1 tablespoon
avocado oil

½ yellow onion, diced

2 garlic cloves, minced

½ red bell pepper, diced

½ yellow bell
pepper, diced

1 (15-ounce) can
black beans, drained
and rinsed

1 (28-ounce) can
diced tomatoes

1 tablespoon
chili powder

2 teaspoons
ground cumin

Salt

Freshly ground
black pepper

2 to 4 zucchinis,
spiralized into zoodles
(3 to 4 cups)

Vegan Sour Cream
(page 85), for garnish

Avocado, diced,
for garnish

Fresh cilantro,
for garnish

1. In a large skillet, heat the avocado oil over medium heat. Add the onion, garlic, red pepper, and yellow pepper and sauté for 4 to 5 minutes, until the onion becomes translucent and soft.
2. Add the black beans, tomatoes with their juices, chili powder, cumin, salt, and pepper. Simmer on low for 15 to 20 minutes, until the veggies are fork-tender.
3. To serve, fill individual bowls halfway with zoodles and the other half with the enchilada mixture. Top with sour cream, avocado, and cilantro.

PER SERVING Calories: 261; Saturated Fat: 6g; Total Fat: 11g; Protein: 11g; Total Carbs: 35g; Fiber: 11g; Sodium: 81mg

Lentil Burrito Bowls

MAKES: 4 SERVINGS / PREP TIME: 10 MINUTES / COOK TIME: 10 MINUTES

GLUTEN-FREE, VEGAN

Lentils and legumes contain protein, vitamins, minerals, and phytonutrients, and they also aid in blood sugar balance and are high in soluble fiber.

2 tablespoons olive oil, divided

½ cup cauliflower rice

¼ cup water (if needed)

1 red bell pepper, diced

1 (8-ounce) package mushrooms, chopped

2 cups cooked brown lentils

¼ red onion, diced

1 teaspoon chili powder

1 teaspoon ground cumin

½ to 1 teaspoon garlic salt

Salt

Freshly ground black pepper

1 head romaine lettuce, chopped

2 tomatoes, diced

1 avocado, diced

Vegan Sour Cream, for topping (page 85; optional)

1. In a large skillet, heat 1 tablespoon of olive oil over medium heat. Add the cauliflower rice and cook for 5 minutes, stirring often, until translucent and soft. If the cauliflower begins to stick, add the water.

2. In another large skillet, heat the remaining 1 tablespoon of olive oil over medium heat. Add the red peppers and mushrooms and sauté for about 5 minutes, until the mushrooms become dark brown and the peppers soften. Add the lentils, onion, chili powder, cumin, and garlic salt and season with salt and pepper. Cook for another 2 minutes, or until the onion becomes soft and translucent.

3. To make the burrito bowls, layer the romaine lettuce, cauliflower rice, and lentil and veggie mixture, and top with the tomato and avocado. Garnish with vegan sour cream (if using).

PER SERVING Calories: 301; Saturated Fat: 2g; Total Fat: 12g; Protein: 15g; Total Carbs: 40g; Fiber: 13g; Sodium: 32mg

Moroccan-Spiced Chickpea Bowls

MAKES: 4-6 SERVINGS / **PREP TIME:** 10 MINUTES / **COOK TIME:** 40 MINUTES

GLUTEN-FREE, NUT-FREE, VEGAN

The garam masala in these bowls offers a host of health benefits.

1 head broccoli, chopped

2 tablespoons avocado oil, divided

½ yellow onion, diced

3 garlic cloves, minced

1 red bell pepper, diced

1½ teaspoons garam masala

½ teaspoon ground coriander

1 teaspoon ground turmeric

1 teaspoon sea salt

½ teaspoon freshly ground black pepper

½ teaspoon paprika

1 teaspoon ground cumin

1 (28-ounce) can diced tomatoes

2 (15.5-ounce) cans chickpeas, drained and rinsed

1. Preheat the oven to 350°F.
2. On a baking sheet, lightly coat the broccoli with 1 tablespoon of avocado oil. Bake for 15 to 20 minutes, until the broccoli becomes charred and fork-tender.
3. Meanwhile, in a large skillet, heat the remaining 1 tablespoon of avocado oil over medium heat and sauté the onion for about 5 minutes. Add the garlic and red peppers and sauté for another 3 to 5 minutes, until the peppers soften.
4. Add the garam masala, coriander, turmeric, salt, pepper, paprika, and cumin and stir until fragrant, about 1 minute.
5. Add the diced tomatoes with their juices and the chickpeas. Simmer on low for 25 minutes.
6. Stir in the broccoli.

INGREDIENT TIP: For a more substantial meal, serve on a bed of warm cauliflower rice.

PER SERVING Calories: 346; Saturated Fat: 1g; Total Fat: 11g; Protein: 15g; Total Carbs: 51g; Fiber: 15g; Sodium: 513mg

Vegan Taco Bowls

MAKES: 4-6 SERVINGS / **PREP TIME:** 15 MINUTES / **COOK TIME:** 5 MINUTES

GLUTEN-FREE, VEGAN

This recipe's "meat" is a complete protein source. Use it in your shepherd's pie, chilis, stews, bowls, and wraps.

4 cups cooked
brown lentils

1½ cup chopped
walnuts

½ teaspoon
onion powder

1 teaspoon dried
oregano

½ teaspoon garlic
powder or salt

2 to 3 teaspoons
ground cumin

1 tablespoon
chili powder

3 to 5 tablespoons
extra-virgin olive
oil, divided

1 tablespoon tamari

1 to 2 cups
mixed greens

1 tomato, finely diced

1 cucumber, sliced

1 avocado, diced

4 scallions, diced

Vegan Sour Cream
(page 85)

1. In a large bowl, mash the lentils and walnuts. Add onion powder, oregano, garlic powder, cumin, chili powder, 2 tablespoons of olive oil, and the tamari and stir to combine. If the mixture is too dry, slowly add olive oil one tablespoon at a time, until the desired consistency is achieved.

2. In a large skillet, heat 1 tablespoon of olive oil over medium heat. Add the lentil and walnut mixture and cook for 5 to 7 minutes, until fragrant.

3. Fill each bowl halfway with the mixed greens, then add the lentil mixture, tomatoes, cucumbers, avocado, and scallions. Top with vegan sour cream.

STORAGE TIP: This taco "meat" mixture freezes well, so if you have leftovers, store in a freezer bag and pull out on a day when you need a quick and easy meal.

PER SERVING Calories: 725; Saturated Fat: 10g; Total Fat: 47g; Protein: 28g; Total Carbs: 59g; Fiber: 24g; Sodium: 315mg

Portobello Fajita Bowls

MAKES: 4–6 SERVINGS / **PREP TIME:** 20 MINUTES, PLUS
30 MINUTES TO MARINATE / **COOK TIME:** 15 MINUTES

GLUTEN-FREE, VEGAN

Portobello mushrooms are a great plant-based protein source. They are nutrient dense, low in calories, and high in disease-fighting antioxidants. If you prefer not to use the marinade below, toss the mushrooms in olive oil and season them with garlic and onion powder.

FOR THE PORTOBELLO MARINADE

2 tablespoons olive oil

2 tablespoons balsamic vinegar

½ teaspoon onion powder

½ teaspoon garlic salt

1 teaspoon chili powder

1 to 2 teaspoons ground cumin

½ teaspoon paprika

TO MAKE THE PORTOBELLO MARINADE

In a small bowl, combine the olive oil, balsamic vinegar, onion powder, garlic salt, chili powder, cumin, and paprika. Mix well.

TO MAKE THE FAJITA BOWLS

1. In a medium bowl with a lid or other lidded container, drizzle the marinade over the mushrooms. Cover and let sit for a minimum of 30 minutes.
2. In a large skillet, heat the avocado oil over medium heat and add the red pepper, yellow pepper, and onion. Cook for 5 minutes, or until the onion is translucent and soft. Transfer to a small bowl and set aside.

FOR THE FAJITA BOWLS

4 to 6 portobello
mushrooms, sliced
into ½-inch strips

1 tablespoon
avocado oil

1 red bell pepper, diced

1 yellow bell
pepper, diced

1 yellow onion, diced

1 cup cooked quinoa

2 cups baby spinach

1 avocado, diced

1 tomato, diced

Vegan Sour Cream
(page 85)

3. In the same skillet, cook the marinated
   mushrooms over medium heat until they are
   softened and have a steak-like appearance,
   and the juices are absorbed, 5 to 10 minutes.
4. To serve, assemble the bowls by dividing
   equally the quinoa, spinach, portobello
   mushrooms, and pepper mixture. Top each
   with avocado, tomato, and vegan sour cream.

STORAGE TIP: Store any leftovers in individual-sized containers in the refrigerator for up to one week; this gives you another meal or two that is prepped and ready to go.

PER SERVING Calories: 336; Saturated Fat: 8g; Total Fat: 24g; Protein: 8g; Total Carbs: 28g; Fiber: 7g; Sodium: 57mg

Vegan Shepherd's Pie with Cauliflower Mash

MAKES: 6 SERVINGS / PREP TIME: 10 MINUTES / COOK TIME: 30 MINUTES

GLUTEN-FREE, NUT-FREE, VEGAN

This cauliflower mash provides vitamin C and potassium. The nutritional yeast supplies B_{12}.

2 tablespoons olive oil, divided

3 garlic cloves, minced, divided

½ yellow onion, diced, divided

1 (8-ounce) package cremini mushrooms

2 tablespoons nutritional yeast (optional)

1 to 2 cups vegetable broth

1½ teaspoons ground cumin

½ teaspoon salt

½ teaspoon freshly ground black pepper

3 to 4 cups cauliflower rice

⅓ cup water

2 cups peas

2 cups cooked brown lentils

1. Preheat the oven to 350°F.
2. In a large skillet, heat 1 tablespoon of olive oil over medium heat. Add 1 minced garlic clove, half of the diced onion, and the mushrooms and cook until the mushrooms are browned, about 5 minutes. Add the nutritional yeast (if using), broth, cumin, salt, and pepper.
3. In another large skillet over medium heat, heat the remaining 1 tablespoon of olive oil, the cauliflower rice, water, and the remaining garlic and onion. Cook until the cauliflower is translucent, 3 to 5 minutes. Transfer to a large bowl and mash.
4. Layer the bottom of a 9-by-11-inch casserole dish with the peas.
5. Mix the lentils into the mushroom mixture and place on top of the peas.
6. Top with the cauliflower mash.
7. Bake for 20 minutes, until heated through.

STORAGE TIP: This recipe can be frozen and then thawed in the refrigerator. Add 10 minutes to the baking time for a total of 30 minutes.

PER SERVING Calories: 188 ; Saturated Fat: 1g; Total Fat: 5g; Protein: 11g; Total Carbs: 26g; Fiber: 9g; Sodium: 260mg

Slow Cooker Barbecue Lentil Chili

MAKES: 4–6 SERVINGS / **PREP TIME:** 10 MINUTES / **COOK TIME:** 8 HOURS

GLUTEN-FREE, VEGAN

This is a great recipe to prep and stick in the freezer. Put all ingredients except for the broth in a large freezer bag. When you're ready to eat the chili, put the bag's contents plus broth into a slow cooker.

4 cups vegetable broth

1 (16-ounce) bag dried red lentils

1 (28-ounce) can diced tomatoes

1 (19-ounce) can 6-bean mix

1 yellow bell pepper, diced

⅓ yellow onion, diced

4 garlic cloves, minced

1 tablespoon chili powder

2 teaspoons ground cumin

¼ cup Homemade Barbecue Sauce (page 80)

Salt

Freshly ground black pepper

Vegan Sour Cream, for garnish (page 85; optional)

1. In a slow cooker, add the broth, lentils, tomatoes with their juices, 6-bean mix, yellow pepper, onion, garlic, chili powder, cumin, and barbecue sauce and season with salt and pepper.
2. Cover and cook on low for 6 to 8 hours, until the lentils are soft.
3. Garnish with vegan sour cream (if using).

COOKING TIP: If you do not have a slow cooker, you can make this recipe in a large pot on the stove. Add the broth, lentils, tomatoes, 6-bean mix, yellow pepper, onion, garlic, chili powder, cumin, and barbecue sauce and season with salt and pepper. Cook on medium-low heat for 1 hour, until the lentils are soft.

PER SERVING Calories: 635; Saturated Fat: 6g; Total Fat: 8g; Protein: 39g; Total Carbs: 102g; Fiber: 43g; Sodium: 212mg

Zoodle Lasagna with Basil Cashew Cheese

MAKES: 6 SERVINGS / **PREP TIME:** 25 MINUTES, PLUS
OVERNIGHT TO SOAK / **COOK TIME:** 40 MINUTES

GLUTEN-FREE, VEGAN

Zucchinis are high in vitamins, minerals, antioxidants, and anti-inflammatory phytonutrients, and they can help regulate blood sugar because they are high in fiber.

FOR THE VEGAN BASIL CASHEW CHEESE

1½ cups cashews, soaked overnight and drained

¼ cup fresh basil

2 garlic cloves, minced

½ teaspoon salt

½ teaspoon freshly ground black pepper

½ to 1 cup unsweetened original almond milk

TO MAKE THE VEGAN BASIL CASHEW CHEESE

1. In a food processor, blend the cashews, basil, garlic, salt, and pepper until smooth.
2. Blend in the almond milk, ½ cup at a time, until you've reached your desired consistency.

TO MAKE THE LASAGNA

1. Preheat the oven to 350°F.
2. Sprinkle the zucchini strips with salt. Let sit for 5 to 10 minutes, then dab with a paper towel to remove the extra water.
3. To assemble the lasagna, cover the bottom of a 9-by-13-inch pan with one-third of the marinara sauce. Add one-third of the zoodles, and half each of the cashew cheese mixture, spinach, mushrooms, and red peppers. Repeat with another layer of the sauce, half of the remaining zoodles, and the remaining cashew cheese, spinach, mushrooms, and red peppers.

FOR THE LASAGNA

4 zucchinis, cut into long, thin lasagna-type "zoodles," divided

1 batch Homemade Marinara Sauce (page 82), divided

2 cups baby spinach, divided

1 (8-ounce) package cremini mushrooms, sliced, divided

1 (12-ounce) jar roasted red peppers, diced, divided

Nutritional yeast, for topping (optional)

4. Finish with the remaining zoodles and marinara sauce on top. Sprinkle with the nutritional yeast (if using).

5. Cover with aluminum foil and bake for 30 minutes. Remove the foil and bake for 10 minutes.

6. Remove from the oven and let sit for 5 to 10 minutes before serving.

INGREDIENT TIP: Zucchini retains a lot of water, so the salting process pulls moisture from the slices and makes the lasagna less watery.

VARIATION TIP: If you have picky eaters who don't enjoy vegetables, you can purée the peppers and spinach and add to the marinara sauce instead—it's a great way to pack the sauce with more nutrients!

PER SERVING Calories: 476; Saturated Fat: 5g; Total Fat: 36g; Protein: 12g; Total Carbs: 33g; Fiber: 8g; Sodium: 703mg

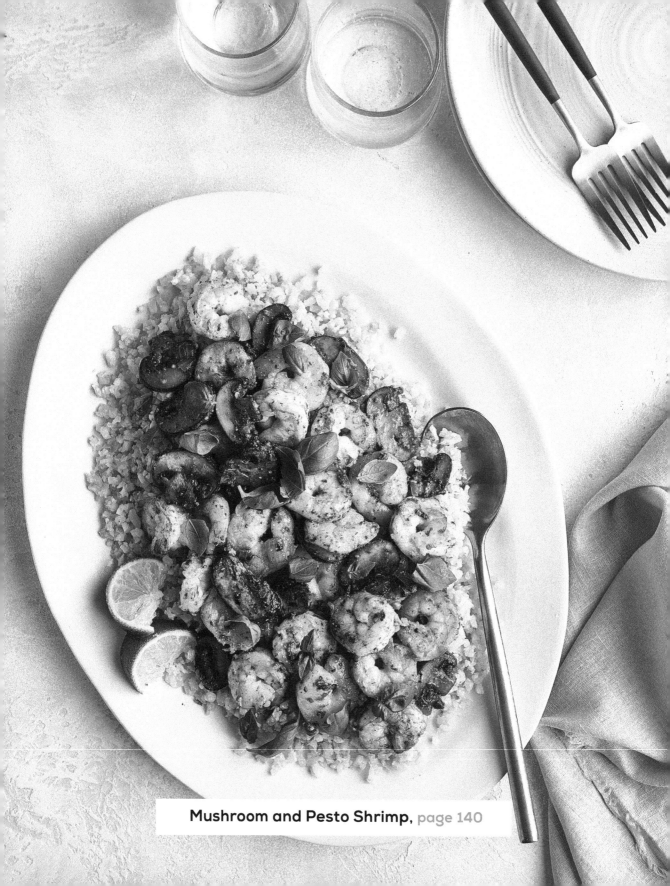

Mushroom and Pesto Shrimp, page 140

9

Seafood Mains

This chapter's fish and shellfish recipes can be prepared quickly. If you like spice, try the Blackened White Fish (page 143) or the Cajun White Fish (page 147). If you want a traditional fish recipe, try the Garlic-Dill White Fish with Asparagus (page 146). The Salmon Cakes with Roasted Red Pepper Drizzle (page 142) can be made during a meal prep session. Individually wrap and freeze them for breakfast, lunch, or dinner. The Garlic Shrimp Zoodles (page 145) is a healthy and delicious substitute for traditional seafood pasta.

Shrimp Buddha Bowls

MAKES: 4 SERVINGS / PREP TIME: 10 MINUTES / COOK TIME: 10 MINUTES

GLUTEN-FREE

To cut this recipe's cook time, I call for precooked shrimp. However, if you want to enhance the flavor and texture of your shrimp, buy them raw and cook them yourself. After rinsing, peeling, and deveining the shrimp, pan-sear them for 2 minutes on each side. You will know when the shrimp are cooked through because they will turn pink.

FOR THE SHRIMP

½ cup almond flour

½ teaspoon onion powder

½ teaspoon garlic powder

½ teaspoon dried oregano

½ teaspoon paprika

Pinch salt

Pinch freshly ground pepper

1 egg, whisked

1 tablespoon coconut oil

30 large cooked shrimp, peeled and deveined (thawed if frozen)

TO MAKE THE SHRIMP

1. In a medium bowl, combine the almond flour, onion powder, garlic powder, oregano, paprika, salt, and pepper.
2. Dip each shrimp in the egg, then coat in the almond flour mixture.
3. In a large skillet, heat the coconut oil over medium heat and cook the shrimp for 1 to 2 minutes on each side, until they are a bit golden.

FOR THE BOWLS

2 cups mixed greens

1 cup cooked quinoa (optional)

20 cherry tomatoes, halved

1 English cucumber, sliced

2 medium carrots, shredded

Roasted Red Pepper Dressing (page 74)

TO MAKE THE BOWLS

1. Divide the mixed greens, quinoa (if using), tomatoes, cucumbers, carrots, and shrimp equally among four bowls.
2. Drizzle each salad with the dressing and toss before serving.

SUBSTITUTION TIP: If you do not eat eggs, you can make a vegan egg wash to coat the shrimp. Take 1 (8-ounce) container of hummus and add water little by little, until the mixture has an egg-like consistency.

PER SERVING Calories: 327; Saturated Fat: 5g; Total Fat: 16g; Protein: 30g; Total Carbs: 17g; Fiber: 3g; Sodium: 316mg

Almond-Crusted Salmon

MAKES: 4 SERVINGS / **PREP TIME:** 5–10 MINUTES / **COOK TIME:** 10 MINUTES

GLUTEN-FREE

Salmon is a great source of omega-3 fatty acids, which help reduce inflammation, potentially improving heart health, brain function, and eye health. Almonds (or almond meal) add antioxidants, protein, vitamin E, calcium, magnesium, and healthy fats.

½ cup almond meal

½ teaspoon garlic salt

½ teaspoon onion powder

Pinch freshly ground black pepper

4 (5-ounce) skinless salmon fillets

1 egg, whisked

1 to 2 tablespoons avocado oil

½ lemon

1. In a small bowl, combine the almond meal, garlic salt, onion powder, and pepper.
2. Dip each salmon fillet into the egg, then coat with the almond mixture and set aside on a plate.
3. In a large skillet, heat the avocado oil over medium heat. Cook the fillets for 3 to 5 minutes, flip, and cook for 3 to 5 minutes more, until the salmon turns whitish in color.
4. Squeeze the lemon juice over the fish before serving.

INGREDIENT TIP: Atlantic salmon is typically farmed, whereas Pacific salmon is primarily wild-caught, which is what you want to aim for when buying fish and seafood. There are five varieties of Pacific salmon in North America: coho, chum, king (chinook), pink, and sockeye.

PER SERVING Calories: 300; Saturated Fat: 3g; Total Fat: 21g; Protein: 26g; Total Carbs: 3g; Fiber: 2g; Sodium: 67mg

Creamy Tuscan Salmon

MAKES: 4 SERVINGS / PREP TIME: 10 MINUTES / COOK TIME: 20 MINUTES

GLUTEN-FREE, NUT-FREE

This recipe contains healthy fats such as omega-3s, and it's high in protein.

2 tablespoons avocado oil, divided

4 (5-ounce) skinless salmon fillets

⅓ yellow onion, diced

4 garlic cloves, minced

1 (8-ounce) package cremini mushrooms, sliced

1 cup halved cherry tomatoes

2 cups chopped spinach

2 roasted red bell peppers, diced

¼ cup nutritional yeast

1 (13.5-ounce) can coconut milk

Salt

Freshly ground black pepper

Fresh parsley, for garnish

1. In a large skillet, heat 1 tablespoon of avocado oil over medium-high heat. Cook the salmon fillets for 4 minutes on each side, until the salmon turns whitish in color. Transfer the fillets to a plate and set aside.
2. In the same skillet, heat the remaining 1 tablespoon of avocado oil over medium heat. Add the onion, garlic, and mushrooms. Sauté for 4 minutes, until the onion is translucent and the mushrooms are soft.
3. Add the cherry tomatoes and spinach and cook for another 2 minutes, until the spinach is wilted.
4. Stir in the red peppers, nutritional yeast, and coconut milk and cook for 5 minutes, or until warm. Add the salmon to the skillet and coat with the sauce.
5. Serve warm and garnish with salt, pepper, and parsley.

SERVING TIP: Serve with cauliflower rice, grilled asparagus, or your favorite veggies.

PER SERVING Calories: 618; Saturated Fat: 29g; Total Fat: 47g; Protein: 39g; Total Carbs: 18g; Fiber: 5g; Sodium: 190mg

Mushroom and Pesto Shrimp

MAKES: 2 SERVINGS / **PREP TIME:** 10 MINUTES / **COOK TIME:** 15 MINUTES

GLUTEN-FREE

This recipe's dairy-free pesto pairs well with chicken or fish. Refrigerate leftover pesto up to one week, or freeze it in ice cube trays up to one month.

FOR THE PESTO

3 cups fresh basil

½ cup nutritional yeast

½ cup olive oil

¼ cup pine nuts or chopped walnuts

2 tablespoons shelled hemp seeds

2 tablespoons freshly squeezed lemon juice

3 garlic cloves

Salt

Freshly ground black pepper

TO MAKE THE PESTO

In a food processor, blend the basil, nutritional yeast, olive oil, pine nuts, hemp seeds, lemon juice, garlic, salt, and pepper until smooth.

TO MAKE THE SHRIMP

1. In a medium bowl, combine the shrimp with ¼ cup of pesto, just enough to coat each shrimp, and set aside to marinate for 25 minutes.
2. Meanwhile, in a large skillet, heat 1 tablespoon of avocado oil over medium heat. Cook the garlic, onion, and mushrooms for about 5 minutes, until the mushrooms are browned. Transfer to a large bowl and set aside.

FOR THE SHRIMP

20 large cooked shrimp, peeled and devined (thawed if frozen)

2 tablespoons avocado oil, divided

2 garlic cloves, minced

½ yellow onion, diced

1 (8-ounce) package mushrooms, sliced

2 cups cauliflower rice

1 lime, cut into wedges, for serving

3. In the same skillet, add the remaining 1 table-spoon of avocado oil and cook the cauliflower rice over medium heat for 5 minutes, until the cauliflower is translucent. Transfer to a medium bowl and set aside.
4. In the same skillet over medium-high heat, add the shrimp and cook for 1 to 2 minutes on each side, until the shrimp turn slightly opaque. Add the mushrooms and remaining pesto and stir to combine.
5. Serve the pesto shrimp over the cauliflower rice. Garnish with fresh lime juice.

COOKING TIP: Thaw frozen, cooked shrimp by running them under cold water. Then, pat dry with a paper towel and remove the tails.

SUBSTITUTION TIP: This recipe also works well with zoodles instead of cauliflower rice.

PER SERVING Calories: 1054; Saturated Fat: 10g; Total Fat: 80g; Protein: 71g; Total Carbs: 25g; Fiber: 10g; Sodium: 556mg

Salmon Cakes with Roasted Red Pepper Drizzle

MAKES: 4-6 CAKES / **PREP TIME:** 10 MINUTES / **COOK TIME:** 25 MINUTES

GLUTEN-FREE

These protein-packed salmon cakes can be cooked and frozen for up to 1 month. Reheat the cakes by baking them in the oven as described below, or pan-fry them until they are heated through, about 4 minutes per side. Serve them with a mixed greens salad.

2 (6-ounce) cans sockeye salmon, drained (or 2 cooked fillets, flaked)

1 egg

1 small red bell pepper, finely diced

1 carrot, grated

1 scallion, finely chopped

2 to 4 tablespoons ground flaxseed

1 garlic clove, minced

½ teaspoon garlic powder

Pinch salt

Pinch freshly ground black pepper

Roasted Red Pepper Dressing (page 74)

Fresh parsley, for garnish (optional)

1. Preheat the oven to 375°F and line a baking sheet with parchment paper.
2. In a large bowl, mix the salmon, egg, red pepper, carrot, scallion, flaxseed, garlic, garlic powder, salt, and pepper.
3. Using your hands, make 4 to 6 cakes, packing tightly to keep them from crumbling. Place on the baking sheet.
4. Bake for 12 minutes, then flip and cook an additional 10 to 12 minutes. The salmon cakes should be slightly browned on the outside.
5. Drizzle with the dressing and garnish with fresh parsley (if using).

PER SERVING Calories: 426; Saturated Fat: 5g; Total Fat: 23g; Protein: 45g; Total Carbs: 11g; Fiber: 3g; Sodium: 216mg

Blackened White Fish

MAKES: 2 SERVINGS / PREP TIME: 10 MINUTES / COOK TIME: 10 MINUTES

GLUTEN-FREE, NUT-FREE

You can easily adjust this recipe's heat level: Omit the cayenne if you prefer less heat, or add a little more paprika, chili powder, or cayenne if you like more heat. Smoked paprika imparts a slightly charred flavor to this fish.

2 teaspoons paprika

½ teaspoon freshly ground black pepper

½ teaspoon garlic powder

½ teaspoon onion powder

½ teaspoon chili powder

½ teaspoon salt

¼ teaspoon dried thyme

⅛ teaspoon cayenne

2 (4- to 6-ounce) skinless basa fillets (or white fish of your choice)

2 tablespoons avocado oil, divided

1. In a small bowl, add the paprika, pepper, garlic powder, onion powder, chili powder, salt, thyme, and cayenne and mix well.
2. Coat the fish fillets in 1 tablespoon of avocado oil. Sprinkle half of the spice mixture on top of the fillets and press the spices into the fish.
3. In a large skillet over medium heat, heat the remaining 1 tablespoon of avocado oil. Place the fish in the pan, spice-side down, and cook for 4 minutes. Season the other side of the fish with the remaining spice mixture.
4. Flip and fry for another 4 minutes.
5. Serve warm.

PER SERVING Calories: 218; Saturated Fat: 2g; Total Fat: 16g; Protein: 17g; Total Carbs: 3g; Fiber: 1g; Sodium: 704mg

Balsamic Reduction Glazed Salmon

MAKES: 2 SERVINGS / PREP TIME: 5 MINUTES / COOK TIME: 30 MINUTES

GLUTEN-FREE, NUT-FREE

Serve this salmon with a side of Roasted Veggie Mix (page 69). Double the amount of balsamic vinegar and place any leftover reduction sauce in a squeeze bottle in the refrigerator. Add the sauce to salads, soups, fish, or chicken.

1 cup balsamic vinegar

2 (5-ounce) skinless salmon fillets

Pinch salt

Pinch freshly ground black pepper

2 tablespoons avocado oil

2 garlic cloves, minced

1. In a small pot over medium-high heat, put the balsamic vinegar and reduce down by 75 percent, periodically stirring. The glaze will become syrupy and thicken in about 20 minutes.
2. Season the salmon fillets with salt and pepper.
3. In a large skillet, heat the avocado oil. Add the garlic and sauté for about 30 seconds, then add the salmon and cook for 4 minutes per side, until the salmon turns whitish in color.
4. Drizzle the salmon with the balsamic reduction sauce to serve.

PER SERVING Calories: 389; Saturated Fat: 5g; Total Fat: 29g; Protein: 28g; Total Carbs: 2g; Fiber: 0g; Sodium: 84mg

Garlic Shrimp Zoodles

MAKES: 4 SERVINGS / **PREP TIME:** 15 MINUTES / **COOK TIME:** 10 MINUTES

GLUTEN-FREE, NUT-FREE

This pasta makes for a quick and easy dinner or lunch. For a different spin on the sauce, add 3 tablespoons of Cashew Cheese Sauce (page 84).

4 tablespoons avocado oil, divided

½ cup chopped broccoli

½ cup chopped cauliflower

½ cup chopped red cabbage

½ red bell pepper, diced

4 garlic cloves, finely minced

30 large cooked shrimp, peeled and deveined (thawed if frozen)

½ tablespoon paprika

Pinch salt

Pinch freshly ground black pepper

2 zucchinis, spiralized into zoodles (about 3 cups)

1½ teaspoons fresh parsley, for garnish

1. In a large skillet, heat 1 tablespoon of avocado oil over medium-high heat. Add the broccoli, cauliflower, red cabbage, and red pepper and sauté for 5 minutes, until tender and slightly golden.
2. Remove from the heat and set aside in a bowl.
3. Heat the remaining 3 tablespoons of avocado oil in the same skillet over medium heat. Add the garlic and cook for 1 minute, until golden and fragrant.
4. Add the shrimp, paprika, salt, and pepper and cook for 1 to 2 minutes on each side, until the shrimp turn pink.
5. Add the zoodles and vegetable mixture to the skillet and mix quickly to combine. Do not overcook—you just want to heat the zoodles.
6. Garnish with parsley and serve warm.

VARIATION TIP: This recipe is versatile when it comes to veggies. Mix it up by adding your favorite veggies or whatever you have in the refrigerator.

PER SERVING Calories: 370; Saturated Fat: 3g; Total Fat: 21g; Protein: 35g; Total Carbs: 12g; Fiber: 3g; Sodium: 366mg

Garlic-Dill White Fish with Asparagus

MAKES: 2 SERVINGS / PREP TIME: 10 MINUTES / COOK TIME: 20 MINUTES

GLUTEN-FREE, NUT-FREE

Bulk up this recipe by adding sweet potato slices or cooked quinoa. Change its flavor by using basil instead of dill.

2 (4- to 6-ounce) skinless basa fillets (or white fish of your choice)

2 tablespoons avocado oil, divided

3 garlic cloves, minced

¼ cup finely chopped fresh dill

¼ teaspoon salt, plus a pinch

¼ teaspoon freshly ground black pepper, plus a pinch

1 lemon, thinly sliced

1 bunch asparagus, ends trimmed

½ teaspoon garlic powder

1. Preheat the oven to 375°F. Line 2 baking sheets with parchment paper.
2. Coat the fish with 1 tablespoon of avocado oil and place on the first baking sheet. Evenly spread the minced garlic over both fillets.
3. Sprinkle the fillets with the fresh dill and season with a pinch of salt and pepper. Place the lemon slices on top of the fillets.
4. Lay the asparagus on the second baking sheet. Coat with the remaining 1 tablespoon of avocado oil and massage the asparagus with your hands to ensure each piece is evenly coated.
5. Sprinkle the asparagus with the garlic powder and ¼ teaspoon each of salt and pepper.
6. Place both baking sheets in the oven and bake for 20 minutes. Serve the fillets warm with the asparagus.

COOKING TIP: You can also wrap the fish and asparagus in foil and grill for 5 minutes.

PER SERVING Calories: 247; Saturated Fat: 2g; Total Fat: 16g; Protein: 20g; Total Carbs: 9g; Fiber: 3g; Sodium: 230mg

Cajun White Fish

MAKES: 2 SERVINGS / **PREP TIME:** 5 MINUTES / **COOK TIME:** 10 MINUTES

GLUTEN-FREE, NUT-FREE

Fish is high in protein and healthy fats, and it is lower in calories than most meats. This recipe will also work with shrimp—simply double or triple the spice mix. Coat the shrimp with an oil or egg wash, season them with the spice mix, and cook them until they turn pink, about 4 minutes.

1 teaspoon paprika

½ teaspoon onion powder

½ teaspoon garlic powder

½ teaspoon red pepper flakes or chili powder

½ teaspoon dried oregano

¼ teaspoon cayenne

¼ teaspoon salt

¼ teaspoon freshly ground black pepper

2 (5-ounce) skinless basa fillets (or white fish of your choice)

2 tablespoons avocado oil, divided

2 garlic cloves, minced

1. In a small bowl, combine the paprika, onion powder, garlic powder, red pepper flakes, oregano, cayenne, salt, and pepper and mix well.
2. Coat the fish fillets with 1 tablespoon of avocado oil and season with half of the spice mixture.
3. In a large skillet, heat the remaining 1 tablespoon of avocado oil over medium heat. Add the garlic and cook until fragrant, 30 seconds to 1 minute. Add the fish, spice-side down, and cook for 4 minutes.
4. While the fish is cooking, coat the top of the fish with the remaining spice mixture. After 4 minutes, flip and cook for another 4 minutes, until the fish is cooked through.

COOKING TIP: The fish can also be baked in the oven at 350°F for 20 to 25 minutes.

PER SERVING Calories: 235; Saturated Fat: 2g; Total Fat: 14g; Protein: 23g; Total Carbs: 3g; Fiber: 1g; Sodium: 292mg

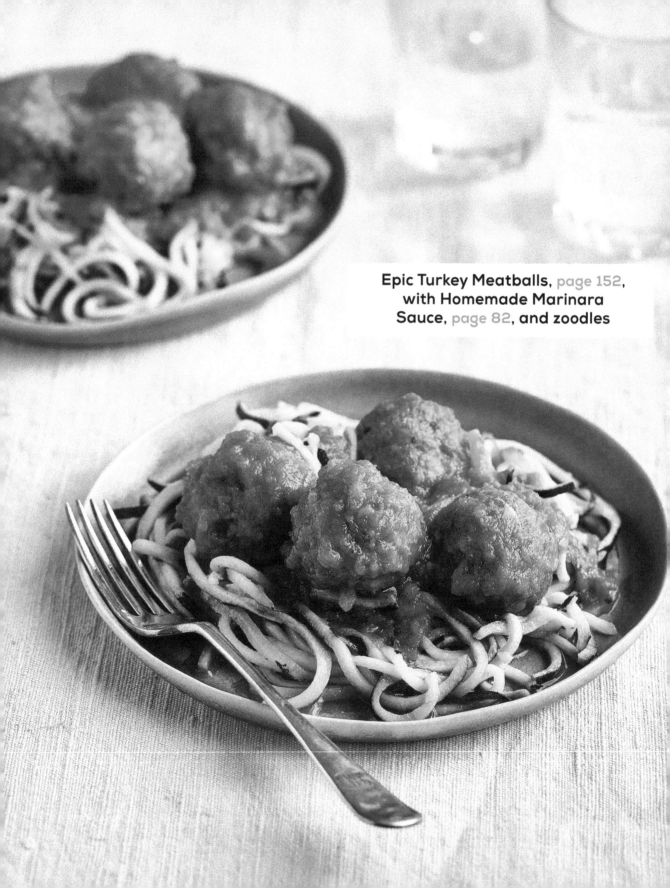

Epic Turkey Meatballs, page 152, with Homemade Marinara Sauce, page 82, **and zoodles**

10

Poultry and Lean Meat Mains

This chapter presents no-fuss, protein-packed chicken and beef recipes. The Cilantro-Lime Chicken with Black Bean Salsa (page 163) and Mexican-Inspired Chicken Casserole (page 155) make for great freezer meals. Thaw them overnight in the refrigerator and pop them in your slow cooker in the morning. Southwest Turkey Chili (page 168) and Cauli Mash Shepherd's Pie (page 160) are comfort foods for cold days. For iron, protein, zinc, vitamin B_{12}, and selenium, try the Zoodle Beef Chow Mein (page 158) or Beef and Cauliflower Rice Stir-Fry (page 166).

Cashew Chicken with Cauliflower Rice

MAKES: 4 SERVINGS / PREP TIME: 10 MINUTES / COOK TIME: 15 MINUTES

GLUTEN-FREE

This recipe is high in protein and low in carbohydrates. Its red peppers are high in vitamins C and A, potassium, and fiber. Vitamin C helps improve immune system function, protein metabolism, and biosynthesis of collagen. It also helps improve the absorption of nonheme iron and has been shown to regenerate antioxidants.

½ cup cashews

2 tablespoons avocado oil, divided

3 to 4 garlic cloves, minced

1 teaspoon minced fresh ginger

¼ medium yellow onion, diced

2 pounds boneless, skinless chicken thighs, cut into 1-inch chunks

1 red bell pepper, diced

1. In a small skillet, toast the cashews over low heat for 1 to 2 minutes, until they lightly brown and become fragrant. Remove from the heat and set aside.
2. In a large skillet, heat 1 tablespoon of avocado oil over medium heat. Add the garlic, ginger, onion, and chicken and cook for 5 minutes, or until the chicken is no longer pink. Add the red pepper, green pepper, tamari, hot sauce, rice vinegar, and sesame oil.
3. Cook for another 2 minutes to reduce the liquid; if you want to thicken the sauce, add the optional tapioca starch.
4. In another large skillet, heat the remaining 1 tablespoon of avocado oil over medium heat. Add the cauliflower rice and cook for 5 minutes, stirring often, until the cauliflower is translucent and soft.

1 green bell
pepper, diced

½ tablespoon tamari
or coconut aminos

½ tablespoon Frank's
RedHot Original sauce

1 tablespoon rice
wine vinegar

1 tablespoon toasted
sesame oil

½ tablespoon tapioca
starch (optional)

2 cups cauliflower rice

2 tablespoons
sesame seeds

Fresh cilantro or
parsley, for garnish

5. To assemble the bowls, use the cauliflower rice as the base and ladle the chicken mixture over it. Top each bowl with the cashews, sesame seeds, and fresh cilantro or parsley.

RECIPE TIP: You can buy cauliflower rice fresh or frozen at most grocery stores. If you are unable to locate it, make your own by grating 1 head of cauliflower with the largest setting on a cheese grater. If you have a food processor you can quickly rice the cauliflower by pulsing until it is the size of rice, about 5 pulses.

INGREDIENT TIP: Tapioca starch is a gluten-free alternative to cornstarch and is used to thicken recipes, but this recipe will work without it if you are unable to find it. Coconut aminos are soy-free but can be hard to find; if you are unable to locate a bottle, use tamari instead, which is a gluten-free soy sauce that can be found in most grocery stores.

PER SERVING Calories: 447; Saturated Fat: 4g; Total Fat: 23g; Protein: 50g; Total Carbs: 13g; Fiber: 4g; Sodium: 497mg

Epic Turkey Meatballs

MAKES: 4 SERVINGS / **PREP TIME:** 10 MINUTES / **COOK TIME:** 25 MINUTES

GLUTEN-FREE

This recipe is very versatile; experiment by adding chopped greens or Homemade Barbecue Sauce (page 80) or by changing the spices—rosemary and sage or a Cajun spice blend will work well. Serve these meatballs with roasted veggies or a fresh salad. You can also pair with them with my Homemade Marinara Sauce (page 82) and zoodles.

1 pound lean ground turkey

1 egg

2 garlic cloves, minced

½ teaspoon Italian seasoning

½ teaspoon paprika

½ teaspoon garlic salt

½ teaspoon onion powder

¼ cup almond flour or gluten-free bread crumbs

1. Preheat the oven to 375°F. Line a baking sheet with parchment paper.
2. In a medium bowl, combine the turkey, egg, garlic, Italian seasoning, paprika, garlic salt, onion powder, and almond flour.
3. Roll the mixture into 1-inch meatballs and place on the baking sheet.
4. Bake for 25 minutes, until the meatballs are cooked through, flipping halfway.
5. Serve warm.

STORAGE TIP: Meatballs freeze well, so you can prepare them ahead of time and freeze for up to 3 months. Store in an airtight container or freezer bag and when you're ready to eat them, thaw in the refrigerator and bake according to recipe directions.

PER SERVING Calories: 169; Saturated Fat: 1g; Total Fat: 5g; Protein: 29g; Total Carbs: 2g; Fiber: 1g; Sodium: 74mg

Easy Cajun Chicken

MAKES: 2 SERVINGS / **PREP TIME:** 5 MINUTES / **COOK TIME:** 20 MINUTES

GLUTEN-FREE, NUT-FREE

The spices in this recipe have great health benefits—paprika supports healthy digestion and has anti-inflammatory properties, and the capsaicin in cayenne helps boost metabolism and reduce hunger. If you like heat, add more spice to this dish.

2 teaspoons paprika

½ teaspoon freshly ground black pepper

½ teaspoon garlic powder

½ teaspoon onion powder

½ teaspoon chili powder

½ teaspoon salt

¼ teaspoon dried thyme

⅛ teaspoon cayenne

2 boneless, skinless chicken breasts

1 tablespoon avocado oil

1. Preheat the oven to 350°F. Line a baking sheet with parchment paper.
2. In a small bowl, add the paprika, pepper, garlic powder, onion powder, chili powder, salt, thyme, and cayenne and mix well.
3. Place the chicken breasts on the baking sheet and coat with the avocado oil. Sprinkle with half of the spice mixture and press onto the chicken breasts. Turn the breasts over and repeat with the remaining spice mixture.
4. Bake for 20 minutes, until the chicken is no longer pink and has an internal temperature of 165°F. Serve warm.

COOKING TIP: I love to serve this dish with a tray of roasted vegetables for a quick and easy lunch. If you want to prep more than 2 servings, simply double or triple the recipe.

SUBSTITUTION TIP: To make this meal vegetarian, simply substitute 2 cups of cooked chickpeas for the chicken.

PER SERVING Calories: 196; Saturated Fat: 1g; Total Fat: 9g; Protein: 27g; Total Carbs: 3g; Fiber: 1g; Sodium: 564mg

Buffalo Turkey Tacos
in Lettuce Wraps

MAKES: 4 SERVINGS / **PREP TIME:** 10 MINUTES / **COOK TIME:** 20 MINUTES

GLUTEN-FREE

If you can't find Frank's RedHot Original sauce, you can substitute any hot sauce that contains no added sugar (check the ingredients list!). If you do not like heat, top the turkey with ¼ cup to ½ cup of Homemade Barbecue Sauce (page 80).

1 tablespoon ghee or vegan butter

¼ to ⅓ cup Frank's RedHot Original sauce

1 tablespoon avocado oil

2 garlic cloves, minced

¼ yellow onion, diced

1 pound lean ground turkey

1 head romaine lettuce, leaves separated

1 red or orange bell pepper, diced (optional)

1 tomato, diced (optional)

Fresh cilantro, for garnish (optional)

Vegan Sour Cream (page 85; optional)

1. In a small pot, melt the ghee over medium heat. Stir in the hot sauce until combined, about 3 minutes.
2. In a large skillet, heat the avocado oil over medium heat. Add the garlic, onion, and turkey and cook for about 15 minutes, or until the turkey is no longer pink.
3. Add the hot sauce to the turkey and stir to coat, then remove from the heat.
4. Assemble the tacos by spooning equal amounts of the buffalo turkey mixture into the romaine lettuce leaves. If using, top with one or more of the red pepper, tomato, fresh cilantro, and vegan sour cream. Serve and enjoy.

PER SERVING Calories: 219; Saturated Fat: 5g; Total Fat: 12g; Protein: 24g; Total Carbs: 6g; Fiber: 0g; Sodium: 147mg

Mexican-Inspired Chicken Casserole

MAKES: 5-6 SERVINGS / **PREP TIME:** 10 MINUTES / **COOK TIME:** 1 HOUR

GLUTEN-FREE

This casserole comes together in a snap.

2 teaspoons
chili powder

1 teaspoon
ground cumin

1 teaspoon
garlic powder

½ teaspoon
onion powder

Pinch salt

Pinch freshly ground
black pepper

1 (28-ounce) can
diced tomatoes

2 garlic cloves, minced

4 boneless, skinless
chicken breasts

1 (15-ounce) can
black beans

½ orange bell
pepper, diced

½ yellow bell
pepper, diced

1 cup cooked quinoa

Vegan Sour Cream
(page 85; optional)

1. Preheat the oven to 375°F.
2. In a small bowl, combine the chili powder, cumin, garlic powder, onion powder, salt, and pepper.
3. In a 9-by-13-inch casserole dish, place the diced tomatoes with their juices and the garlic in the bottom. Add the spice mixture and stir to combine.
4. Place the chicken breasts on top; do not overlap them.
5. Add the black beans, orange pepper, and yellow pepper and stir all the ingredients to coat the chicken.
6. Bake for 40 minutes, until the chicken has an internal temperature of 165°F. Remove from the oven and shred the chicken with a fork.
7. To serve, place the chicken and quinoa in a bowl. If using, garnish with vegan sour cream, if using.

PER SERVING Calories: 417; Saturated Fat: 1g; Total Fat: 5g; Protein: 40g; Total Carbs: 54g; Fiber: 12g; Sodium: 102mg

Teriyaki Chicken Bowls

MAKES: 6 SERVINGS / **PREP TIME:** 15 MINUTES / **COOK TIME:** 25 MINUTES

GLUTEN-FREE, NUT-FREE

This recipe uses apple butter to add sweetness to the teriyaki sauce.

⅓ cup low-sodium tamari

1 tablespoon toasted sesame oil

½ tablespoon rice vinegar

1 tablespoon Apple Butter (page 86)

2 tablespoons tapioca starch

2 tablespoons avocado oil, divided

3 garlic cloves, minced

½ yellow onion, diced

2 pounds boneless skinless chicken thighs, cut into 1-inch chunks

4 cups chopped broccoli

1 yellow bell pepper, diced

1 red bell pepper, diced

2 cups cauliflower rice

Sesame seeds, for garnish

1. To make the teriyaki sauce, in a small bowl add the tamari, sesame oil, rice vinegar, apple butter, and tapioca starch. Stir well to combine.
2. In a large skillet, heat 1 tablespoon of avocado oil over medium heat. Add the garlic and onion and sauté for 1 to 2 minutes, then add the chicken and cook for 5 to 8 minutes, until no longer pink.
3. Add the broccoli, yellow pepper, and red pepper to the skillet and cook for 3 to 5 minutes, until tender.
4. Add the teriyaki sauce and cook for 3 to 5 minutes, until the sauce thickens and the chicken and vegetables are evenly coated.
5. In a medium skillet, heat the remaining 1 tablespoon of avocado oil over medium heat. Add the cauliflower rice and cook for 5 minutes, until soft and translucent.
6. To serve, spoon the cauliflower rice into bowls, top with the teriyaki chicken, and garnish with sesame seeds.

COOKING TIP: Tapioca starch is used instead of cornstarch as it is gluten-free and corn-free. It's great for helping to thicken up sauces.

PER SERVING Calories: 415; Saturated Fat: 3g; Total Fat: 17g; Protein: 51g; Total Carbs: 18g; Fiber: 5g; Sodium: 943mg

Chicken and Veggie Kabobs

MAKES: 4–6 KABOBS / **PREP TIME:** 10 MINUTES, PLUS 30 MINUTES
TO MARINATE / **COOK TIME:** 20 MINUTES

GLUTEN-FREE, NUT-FREE

This recipe is easy to change up by using shrimp or beef instead of chicken.

Balsamic Dressing
(page 78)

4 boneless, skinless
chicken breasts, cut
into bite-size pieces

1 red bell pepper,
cut into squares

1 yellow bell pepper,
cut into squares

1 orange bell pepper,
cut into squares

1 red onion, cut into
square chunks

1 pint cherry tomatoes

2 zucchinis, sliced
into 2-inch chunks

1 (8-ounce) package
mushrooms

1. Preheat the grill to 375°F to 400°F. Soak wooden skewers in water for 15 minutes to prevent them from burning on the grill. You can also use metal skewers.
2. In a medium bowl, pour the dressing over the chicken. Marinate in the refrigerator for 30 minutes.
3. Assemble the kabobs by alternating the veggies with the chicken to fill each skewer.
4. Grill for about 5 minutes on each side, until the chicken is no longer pink.
5. Transfer the kabobs to a plate and serve hot.

COOKING TIP: You can also bake these chicken skewers in the oven. Preheat the oven to 425°F. Place the skewers on baking sheets lined with parchment paper and bake for 10 to 15 minutes, then flip and bake for another 10 to 15 minutes, until the chicken is no longer pink.

SUBSTITUTION TIP: Replace the chicken with more roasted vegetables or roasted sweet potato for a vegetarian version.

PER SERVING Calories: 349; Saturated Fat: 2g; Total Fat: 16g; Protein: 31g; Total Carbs: 21g; Fiber: 5g; Sodium: 123mg

Zoodle Beef Chow Mein

MAKES: 2-4 SERVINGS / **PREP TIME:** 15 MINUTES / **COOK TIME:** 15 MINUTES

GLUTEN-FREE, NUT-FREE

This recipe works with any type of steak. If you are not a fan of steak, you can substitute chicken or shrimp. Or you can make this dish vegan; simply add your favorite vegan protein source and follow the recipe below.

2.5 tablespoons tamari

2 teaspoons
rice vinegar

1 tablespoon olive oil

1 (8-ounce) flank
steak, thinly sliced
against the grain

½ yellow onion,
finely chopped

1 inch fresh
ginger, minced

2 garlic cloves, minced

1 red bell pepper,
chopped

1 large carrot, shredded

1 cup shredded
red cabbage

¼ cup snap peas,
cut in half

2 medium zucchinis,
spiralized (about
3 cups)

1. In a medium bowl, combine the tamari and rice vinegar and set aside.
2. In a large skillet, heat the olive oil over medium heat. Add the steak, onion, ginger, and garlic and sauté until the steak is cooked to your liking, then remove from the skillet and set aside.
3. In the same skillet over medium heat, add the red pepper, carrots, cabbage, and snap peas and cook for 2 minutes.
4. Add the tamari sauce, zoodles, and steak. Cook for another 2 minutes or until the veggies are soft and the mixture is well incorporated.

INGREDIENT TIP: If you do not have a spiralizer, you can use 3 cups of pre-spiralized zoodles from the grocery store.

PER SERVING Calories: 377; Saturated Fat: 1g; Total Fat: 18g; Protein: 32g; Total Carbs: 24g; Fiber: 7g; Sodium: 1312mg

Spinach and Feta Turkey Burgers

MAKES: 4 BURGERS / **PREP TIME:** 10 MINUTES / **COOK TIME:** 10 MINUTES

GLUTEN-FREE, NUT-FREE

Spinach provides protein, iron, potassium, magnesium, vitamin B$_6$, and folic acid as well as the antioxidant vitamin E, which helps protect against the free radical damage that occurs when we convert the food we eat into energy.

1 pound lean ground turkey

1 egg

½ cup chopped spinach

4 ounces dairy-free feta cheese, crumbled

½ teaspoon paprika

½ teaspoon garlic salt

½ teaspoon onion powder

¼ to ½ cup gluten-free bread crumbs

1 tablespoon avocado oil

Homemade Barbecue Sauce (page 80; optional)

1. Add the ground turkey, egg, spinach, feta cheese, paprika, garlic salt, onion powder, and the bread crumbs to a medium-size bowl and mix to combine.
2. Form 4 patties.
3. In a large skillet, heat the avocado oil over medium heat. Fry the burgers for about 4 minutes on each side, until cooked through.
4. Serve the burgers with homemade barbecue sauce (if using).

COOKING TIP: These burgers are great on the grill, too. Heat the grill and cook for 10 minutes, flipping halfway through. The burgers are done when they're golden brown and a thermometer registers an internal temperature of 165°F.

PER SERVING Calories: 283; Saturated Fat: 6g; Total Fat: 13g; Protein: 34g; Total Carbs: 8g; Fiber: 1g; Sodium: 464mg

Cauli Mash Shepherd's Pie

MAKES: 4-6 SERVINGS / PREP TIME: 10 MINUTES / COOK TIME: 35 MINUTES

GLUTEN-FREE, NUT-FREE

An English dish, shepherd's pie is traditionally made with meat, gravy, and vegetables and is topped with mashed potatoes. This healthier version features lean turkey and ditches the gravy for broth.

2 tablespoons
avocado oil, divided

2 to 3 garlic
cloves, minced

½ yellow onion, diced

1 pound lean
ground turkey

1 cup vegetable,
chicken, or beef broth

3 tablespoons
nutritional yeast

1 teaspoon tamari

½ teaspoon salt

½ teaspoon freshly
ground black pepper

3 to 4 cups
cauliflower rice

1 to 2 cups peas
(fresh or frozen)

1. Preheat the oven to 350°F.
2. In a large skillet, heat 1 tablespoon of avocado oil over medium heat. Add the garlic, onion, and turkey and cook until the meat is browned and cooked through, about 7 minutes. Add the broth, nutritional yeast, tamari, salt, and pepper.
3. In another large skillet, heat the remaining 1 tablespoon of avocado oil. Add the cauliflower rice and cook until translucent, about 5 minutes.
4. Remove from the heat and place in a large bowl. Blend with an immersion blender until the mixture resembles mashed potatoes.
5. Pour enough peas into a 9-by-11-inch casserole dish to cover the bottom.
6. Spread the meat mixture on top of the peas.
7. Top the meat mixture with the cauliflower mash and sprinkle with salt and pepper.
8. Bake for 20 minutes, until heated throughout.

COOKING TIP: If you do not own an immersion blender, you can mash cauliflower rice with a handheld potato masher instead.

PER SERVING Calories: 277; Saturated Fat: 2g; Total Fat: 13g; Protein: 28g; Total Carbs: 14g; Fiber: 5g; Sodium: 482mg

Coconut Chicken Curry

MAKES: 6 SERVINGS / **PREP TIME:** 10 MINUTES / **COOK TIME:** 25 MINUTES

GLUTEN-FREE, NUT-FREE

This recipe works well with a wide range of vegetables. If you have a sweet potato, leftover broccoli, or red peppers, add them to the recipe to increase the amount of nutrients in your meal.

2 tablespoons avocado oil, divided

½ yellow onion, diced

4 garlic cloves, minced

2 pounds boneless, skinless chicken thighs or breasts, cut into bite-size pieces

2 cups cauliflower rice

2 tablespoons curry powder

1 teaspoon ground turmeric

1 teaspoon garam masala

1 teaspoon ground cumin

1 to 2 cups chopped spinach

Pinch salt

Pinch freshly ground black pepper

1½ (13.5-ounce) cans coconut milk

1. In a large skillet, heat 1 tablespoon of avocado oil over medium heat. Add the onion, garlic, and chicken and cook until the onion softens and the meat is cooked through, about 6 minutes.
2. In another skillet, heat the remaining 1 tablespoon of avocado oil over medium heat. Cook the cauliflower rice for about 5 minutes, until soft and translucent.
3. Once the chicken is cooked through, add the curry powder, turmeric, garam masala, cumin, spinach, salt, and pepper and stir for 30 seconds until the chicken is coated and the spinach starts to wilt.
4. Add the coconut milk and stir. Continue to cook on low for 5 to 10 minutes or longer to allow the flavors to combine.
5. Serve the curry over the cauliflower rice.

PER SERVING Calories: 613; Saturated Fat: 28g; Total Fat: 41g; Protein: 57g; Total Carbs: 11g; Fiber: 3g; Sodium: 199mg

Peanut Chicken Tacos in Lettuce Wraps

MAKES: 4 SERVINGS / **PREP TIME:** 10 MINUTES / **COOK TIME:** 10 MINUTES

GLUTEN-FREE

Traditional peanut butter contains added sugar, but all-natural peanut butter contains just roasted peanuts. It also contains protein, phosphorus, potassium, niacin, vitamin B_6, zinc, and magnesium. Magnesium alone plays a role in more than 300 of the body's chemical processes.

1 tablespoon avocado oil

2 garlic cloves, minced

⅓ yellow onion, diced

4 boneless, skinless chicken breasts, cut into bite-size chunks

2 medium carrots, peeled and shredded

1 cup finely chopped red cabbage

1 batch Peanut Curry Sauce (page 83)

1 head romaine lettuce, leaves separated

¼ cup chopped peanuts, for topping (optional)

Fresh cilantro, for garnish

Freshly squeezed lime juice, for garnish

1. In a large skillet, heat the avocado oil over medium heat. Add the garlic, onion, and chicken and cook for 5 to 7 minutes, stirring frequently, until the chicken is cooked through.
2. Add the carrots and red cabbage and cook for 1 to 2 minutes.
3. Add half of the peanut curry sauce to the chicken and veggie mixture. Stir to coat evenly, cook for 1 minute, and remove from the heat. If you like saucier tacos, add more sauce to your liking.
4. Assemble the tacos by spooning the chicken mixture into the lettuce wraps. Garnish with chopped peanuts (if using), cilantro, and lime juice.

PER SERVING Calories: 392; Saturated Fat: 2g; Total Fat: 20g; Protein: 37g; Total Carbs: 19g; Fiber: 3g; Sodium: 608mg

Cilantro-Lime Chicken with Black Bean Salsa

MAKES: 6 SERVINGS / PREP TIME: 10 MINUTES / COOK TIME: 4–8 HOURS

GLUTEN-FREE, NUT-FREE

Cilantro is a great source of antioxidants.

2 pounds boneless, skinless chicken thighs

1 (15-ounce) can black beans, drained and rinsed

1 orange bell pepper, diced

1 yellow bell pepper, diced

1 red bell pepper, diced

½ yellow onion, diced

2 garlic cloves, minced

2 tablespoons freshly squeezed lime juice

3 tablespoons chopped fresh cilantro

2 tablespoons chili powder

1½ teaspoons ground cumin

½ teaspoon paprika

½ teaspoon onion powder

Pinch salt

Pinch black pepper

Place the chicken, black beans, orange pepper, yellow pepper, red pepper, onion, garlic, lime juice, cilantro, chili powder, cumin, paprika, onion powder, salt, and pepper in a slow cooker, and cook on high for 4 hours or low for 7 to 8 hours, until the chicken is cooked through.

COOKING TIP: If you do not have a slow cooker, you can turn this into a casserole. Bake at 350°F for 40 minutes, until the chicken is cooked through.

PER SERVING Calories: 407; Saturated Fat: 2g; Total Fat: 11g; Protein: 52g; Total Carbs: 29g; Fiber: 9g; Sodium: 244mg

Red Thai-Inspired Coconut Curry Chicken Soup

MAKES: 4-6 SERVINGS / **PREP TIME:** 10 MINUTES / **COOK TIME:** 4-8 HOURS

GLUTEN-FREE, NUT-FREE

This dish will come out great if cooked on high, but I find that letting the ingredients cook on low for several extra hours allows the flavors to deepen.

2 garlic cloves, minced

1 inch fresh ginger, shredded or minced

4 boneless, skinless chicken breasts, cut into 1-inch chunks

4 cups vegetable broth

3 tablespoons red curry paste

1½ (13.5-ounce) cans coconut milk

3-inch lemongrass (optional)

1 red bell pepper, diced

2 medium carrots, peeled and chopped

2 to 3 cups chopped spinach or kale

1. Place the garlic, ginger, chicken, broth, curry paste, coconut milk, lemongrass (if using), pepper, and carrots in a slow cooker.
2. Cover and cook on high 4 hours or low for 7 to 8 hours.
3. Add the spinach 10 minutes before serving.

INGREDIENT TIP: If using the lemongrass, chop off the ends and use the bottom 3 inches only. Peel off the tough outer layer, then smash with a meat tenderizer or the bottom of a bottle to release the fragrant oils. Place the entire piece in the slow cooker and remove before serving.

PER SERVING Calories: 534; Saturated Fat: 31g; Total Fat: 39g; Protein: 30g; Total Carbs: 21g; Fiber: 5g; Sodium: 899mg

Pesto-Stuffed Chicken

MAKES: 4 SERVINGS / **PREP TIME:** 15 MINUTES / **COOK TIME:** 30 MINUTES

GLUTEN-FREE

The star of this dish is the dairy-free pesto, and the star ingredient of the pesto is basil. Basil has many health benefits; it is an excellent source of vitamins (K, C, and A), manganese, and iron.

FOR THE PESTO

3 cups fresh basil

½ cup nutritional yeast

½ cup olive oil

¼ cup pine nuts
or walnuts

2 tablespoons shelled
hemp seeds

2 tablespoons freshly
squeezed lemon juice

3 garlic cloves

Pinch salt

Pinch freshly ground
black pepper

FOR THE CHICKEN

4 boneless, skinless
chicken breasts

1 tablespoon
avocado oil

Pinch salt

Pinch freshly ground
black pepper

TO MAKE THE PESTO

In a food processor, blend the basil, nutritional yeast, olive oil, pine nuts, hemp seeds, lemon juice, garlic, salt, and pepper until smooth, about 1 minute.

TO MAKE THE CHICKEN

1. Preheat the oven to 350°F. Line a baking sheet with parchment paper.
2. Cut slits in the sides of the chicken breast, making a pocket in each breast, and place on the baking sheet. Coat the breasts with the avocado oil and sprinkle with salt and pepper.
3. Spoon the pesto into the pockets and lightly coat the outsides. Secure the breasts using toothpicks.
4. Cover with foil and bake until the chicken is cooked through, about 30 minutes.

PER SERVING Calories: 507; Saturated Fat: 5g; Total Fat: 40g; Protein: 34g; Total Carbs: 6g; Fiber: 3g; Sodium: 78mg

Beef and Cauliflower Rice Stir-Fry

MAKES: 4 SERVINGS / **PREP TIME:** 15 MINUTES / **COOK TIME:** 15 MINUTES

GLUTEN-FREE, NUT-FREE

Why cauliflower rice? One cup of cauliflower rice has 25 calories, 4 grams of carbs, 3 grams of fiber, and 3 grams of protein, whereas one cup of rice comes in at 205 calories, 45 grams of carbs, not even one gram of fiber, and 4 grams of protein. This stir-fry uses beef, an excellent source of protein, iron, zinc, and vitamin B_{12}. If you do not eat steak, replace it with chicken, turkey, or pork chops.

FOR THE SAUCE

¼ cup tamari or coconut aminos

2 to 3 tablespoons water

2 tablespoons rice vinegar

1 tablespoon toasted sesame oil

1 teaspoon grated fresh ginger

TO MAKE THE SAUCE

Add the tamari, water, rice vinegar, sesame oil, and ginger to a small bowl and whisk until well combined. If mixture is too thick, add more water 1 tablespoon at a time until the desired consistency is achieved.

FOR THE STIR-FRY

2 tablespoons
avocado oil, divided

1 (8-ounce) flank
steak, thinly sliced
against the grain

½ medium yellow
onion, diced

2 garlic cloves, minced

1 teaspoon grated
fresh ginger

2 medium carrots,
peeled and shredded

1 cup broccoli florets

1 red bell pepper, diced

1 cup shredded
red cabbage

4 cups cauliflower rice

Fresh cilantro,
for garnish

2 tablespoons
sesame seeds

TO MAKE THE STIR-FRY

1. In a large skillet, heat 1 tablespoon of avocado oil over medium heat. Add the flank steak, onion, garlic, and ginger. Cook for 5 to 7 minutes, until the beef is cooked to your liking. Set aside in a bowl.

2. In the same skillet, heat the remaining 1 tablespoon of avocado oil over medium heat. Add the carrots, broccoli, red pepper, and red cabbage. Cook for about 2 minutes, until the veggies have softened.

3. Add the cauliflower rice and cook for another 5 minutes. Add the beef and sauce and stir to combine.

4. To serve, garnish with fresh cilantro and sesame seeds.

PER SERVING Calories: 298; Saturated Fat: 2g; Total Fat: 18g; Protein: 19g; Total Carbs: 17g; Fiber: 6g; Sodium: 961mg

Southwest Turkey Chili

MAKES: 4-6 SERVINGS / PREP TIME: 15 MINUTES / COOK TIME: 30 MINUTES

GLUTEN-FREE

This recipe may look complicated because it has many ingredients, but it's actually quick and easy to make. Simply toss all the ingredients in a pot or a slow cooker and let them simmer. The result is a chili packed with nutrients. Turkey and black beans contain protein, and beans contain iron and fiber and can help with blood sugar regulation.

1 tablespoon avocado oil

½ cup finely chopped yellow onion

2 garlic cloves minced

1 pound lean ground turkey

4 cups chicken broth

1 (28-ounce) can diced tomatoes

1 (15-ounce) can black beans drained and rinsed

1 (4-ounce) can diced green chiles, drained

½ yellow bell pepper, diced

½ orange bell pepper, diced

1 tablespoon chili powder

1 teaspoon ground cumin

½ teaspoon onion powder

½ teaspoon paprika

¼ teaspoon cayenne

Pinch salt

Pinch freshly ground black pepper

Fresh cilantro, for garnish (optional)

Diced avocado, for garnish (optional)

Vegan Sour Cream, for garnish (page 85; optional)

1. In a large pot, heat the avocado oil over medium-high heat. Add the onion, garlic, and turkey. Cook until the onion softens and the turkey is cooked through, about 7 minutes.
2. Add the broth, tomatoes with their juices, black beans, chiles, yellow pepper, orange pepper, chili powder, cumin, onion powder, paprika, cayenne, salt, and pepper. Bring to a boil, then turn the heat to low and simmer for 20 minutes.
3. Serve in bowls and, if using, garnish with cilantro, avocado, or vegan sour cream.

PER SERVING Calories: 449; Saturated Fat: 3g; Total Fat: 15g; Protein: 35g; Total Carbs: 50g; Fiber: 18g; Sodium: 693mg

Grilled Chicken Bruschetta Bowls

MAKES: 3-4 SERVINGS / **PREP TIME:** 10 MINUTES, PLUS
30 MINUTES TO CHILL / **COOK TIME:** 20 MINUTES

GLUTEN-FREE, NUT-FREE

Fresh tomatoes and basil add a ton of flavor to this chicken bowl. Bruschetta is traditionally an Italian antipasto (starter dish) that is served on crusty bread. This healthier version is served with a protein (chicken) and greens.

FOR THE BRUSCHETTA

4 large tomatoes

1 garlic clove, minced

½ cup chopped arugula

¼ cup fresh basil

¼ cup olive oil

1 tablespoon balsamic vinegar

Pinch salt

Pinch freshly ground black pepper

TO MAKE THE BRUSCHETTA

In a medium bowl, add the tomatoes, garlic, arugula, basil, olive oil, balsamic vinegar, salt, and pepper. Marinate in the refrigerator for 30 minutes or longer.

TO ROAST THE CHICKEN

1. Preheat the oven to 350°F. Line a baking sheet with parchment paper.
2. Place the breasts on the baking sheet and rub with the avocado oil and salt and pepper.
3. Bake for 20 minutes, until the chicken reaches an internal temperature of 165°F. Cut into bite-size pieces.

FOR THE ROASTED CHICKEN

2 boneless, skinless chicken breasts

1 tablespoon avocado oil

Pinch salt

Pinch freshly ground black pepper

FOR THE BOWLS

2 to 3 cups arugula or mixed greens

1 cucumber, chopped

1 avocado, diced

Balsamic Dressing (page 78)

TO ASSEMBLE THE BOWLS

In each bowl, combine the mixed greens, chicken, cucumber, bruschetta mixture, and avocado. Drizzle with the balsamic dressing.

PER SERVING Calories: 579; Saturated Fat: 7g; Total Fat: 48g; Protein: 22g; Total Carbs: 22g; Fiber: 7g; Sodium: 103mg

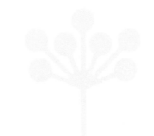

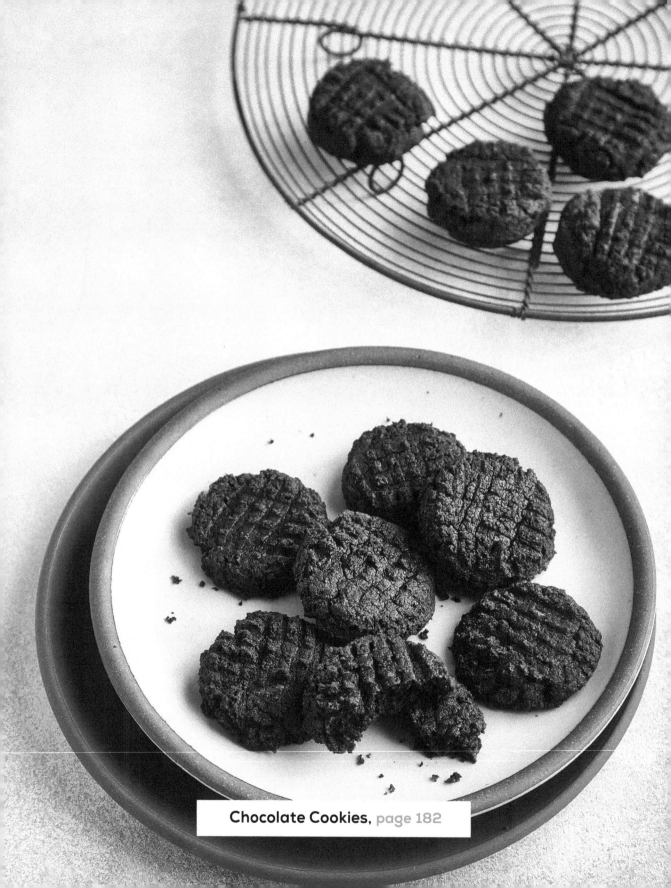

Chocolate Cookies, page 182

11

Desserts

This chapter is heavy on balls and bars that fuel your body with nutrients, healthy proteins, and fats to keep you fuller longer. At the beginning of each week, make one to two batches of one of the balls or bars and store them in the refrigerator. Most of the balls and bars require no baking and take less than 10 minutes to make.

No-Bake Lemon Cake Balls

MAKES: 12–14 BALLS / **PREP TIME:** 10 MINUTES

GLUTEN-FREE, VEGAN

Lemons are a rich source of vitamin C, which promotes the body's immune-boosting abilities. Lemons also aid in liver detoxification by encouraging bile formation to carry toxins away from the liver. When you do a sugar detox, you are looking to avoid sugar first and foremost, but you also want to give your liver a break from having to process chemicals.

1 cup oat or almond flour

⅔ cup unsweetened coconut flakes

¼ cup vegan protein powder

3 tablespoons freshly squeezed lemon juice

2 tablespoons Apple Butter (page 86)

1 teaspoon pure vanilla extract

1. In a large bowl, add the oat flour, coconut flakes, protein powder, lemon juice, apple butter, and vanilla and mix by hand. If the mixture is too dry, add a little more apple butter.
2. Roll into 1-inch balls and serve.

INGREDIENT TIP: You can make your own oat flour by blending gluten-free oats in a food processor. If you do not want to use protein powder, you can substitute ¼ cup of ground flaxseed or ¼ cup of hemp hearts.

STORAGE TIP: Store in an airtight container in the refrigerator for up to one week, or freeze for up to one month.

PER SERVING Calories: 87; Saturated Fat: 4g; Total Fat: 7g; Protein: 3g; Total Carbs: 3g; Fiber: 2g; Sodium: 9mg

Chocolate Protein Donuts

MAKES: 6 DONUTS / PREP TIME: 5 MINUTES / BAKE TIME: 15 MINUTES

GLUTEN-FREE, VEGETARIAN

These donuts are nutritious, not just delicious. During the holidays you can make them festive by topping them with melted dairy-free chocolate.

1 tablespoon coconut oil, melted, plus more for the pan

½ cup almond flour

¼ cup vegan chocolate protein powder

3 tablespoons all-natural almond butter

¼ cup unsweetened applesauce

1 egg

1 teaspoon baking powder

Pinch salt

1. Preheat the oven to 350°F. Lightly grease a donut tray with coconut oil.
2. In a medium bowl, mix the coconut oil, almond flour, protein powder, almond butter, applesauce, egg, baking powder, and salt until combined.
3. Spoon the batter into the donut tray and bake until browned, 12 to 15 minutes.
4. Let cool for 5 minutes, remove the donuts from the tray, and serve.

STORAGE TIP: Store in an airtight container in the refrigerator for up to four days or freeze for up to two weeks.

PER SERVING Calories: 126; Saturated Fat: 3g; Total Fat: 9g; Protein: 7g; Total Carbs: 4g; Fiber: 2g; Sodium: 75mg

Creamy Chocolate Protein Pops

MAKES: 6 POPS / PREP TIME: 5 MINUTES, PLUS 3 HOURS TO FREEZE

GLUTEN-FREE, VEGAN

This recipe requires an ice pop mold with sticks; this inexpensive tool can be purchased online. If you don't want to add protein powder, simply substitute 2 additional tablespoons of cacao powder.

1 cup unsweetened vanilla almond milk

¼ cup vegan chocolate protein powder

2 tablespoons cacao powder

1 tablespoon almond butter

1. In a blender, blend the almond milk, protein powder, cacao powder, and almond butter until well combined.
2. Divide the mixture evenly among 6 ice pop molds. Place the ice pop sticks in the centers and freeze for at least 3 hours, or overnight. Serve and enjoy.

VARIATION TIP: If you'd prefer sweeter pops, add 1 frozen banana to the mixture before freezing.

PER SERVING Calories: 58; Saturated Fat: 1g; Total Fat: 3g; Protein: 6g; Total Carbs: 4g; Fiber: 2g; Sodium: 77mg

Pumpkin Protein Balls

MAKES: 12–15 BALLS / PREP TIME: 5 MINUTES

GLUTEN-FREE, NUT-FREE, VEGAN

These delicious protein balls use Apple Butter (page 86) as a binder and to add a little natural sweetness. Sweeter options, like pure honey, would also work if you're not on the detox, but the lower-sugar apple butter is preferable.

1 cup gluten-free rolled oats

¼ cup vegan vanilla protein powder

⅓ cup canned pumpkin purée (not pumpkin pie filling)

1 tablespoon hemp hearts

2 tablespoons Apple Butter (page 86)

1 teaspoon pumpkin pie spice

1 teaspoon ground cinnamon

⅓ cup unsweetened coconut flakes (optional)

1. In a large bowl, mix the oats, protein powder, pumpkin purée, hemp hearts, apple butter, pumpkin pie spice, and cinnamon until well combined.
2. Roll into 12 to 15 balls.
3. Coat the balls in coconut flakes (if using), before serving.

INGREDIENT TIP: You can also add cacao nibs or dairy-free chocolate chips to this recipe.

STORAGE TIP: Store in an airtight container in the refrigerator for up to four days or freeze for up to one month.

PER SERVING Calories: 45; Saturated Fat: 0g; Total Fat: 1g; Protein: 3g; Total Carbs: 6g; Fiber: 1g; Sodium: 22mg

Blueberry Oatmeal Muffin Cups

MAKES: 12 MUFFINS / **PREP TIME:** 5 MINUTES / **COOK TIME:** 15 MINUTES

GLUTEN-FREE, NUT-FREE, VEGETARIAN

These oat cups make an easy grab-and-go breakfast, snack, or dessert. Blueberries are loaded with antioxidants, and oats help regulate blood sugar and reduce inflammation.

2 bananas

1 teaspoon pure vanilla extract

1 egg

¼ cup unsweetened applesauce

1½ cups gluten-free rolled oats

½ cup vegan vanilla protein powder or ½ cup oat flour

1 tablespoon ground flaxseed

2 teaspoons baking powder

½ cup blueberries, fresh or frozen

1. Preheat the oven to 375°F. Line a muffin tin with muffin liners.
2. In a large bowl, mash the bananas until they are smooth. Add the vanilla, egg, and applesauce and stir to combine.
3. In another large bowl, combine the oats, protein powder, flaxseed, and baking powder.
4. Mix the wet ingredients into the dry ingredients and stir until incorporated. Stir in the blueberries.
5. Fill each muffin cup halfway to three-quarters full.
6. Bake for 15 minutes, until the muffins are cooked through and slightly golden.
7. Allow the muffins to cool for a few minutes before serving.

SUBSTITUTION TIP: You can swap out the blueberries for dairy-free chocolate chips or chopped nuts.

PER SERVING Calories: 92; Saturated Fat: 0g; Total Fat: 2g; Protein: 6g; Total Carbs: 14g; Fiber: 2g; Sodium: 49mg

Chocolate Avocado Mousse

MAKES: 2–3 SERVINGS / **PREP TIME:** 10 MINUTES

GLUTEN-FREE, VEGAN

Avocados are a nutrient-dense superfood. They have anti-inflammatory properties and are a great source of vitamins C and E, which help boost immune system function. They also provide healthy fats, which aid in lubricating joints and moisturizing skin. Still another health benefit: The fiber content of avocados helps regulate blood sugar levels.

1½ cups unsweetened vanilla almond milk

½ avocado

1 frozen banana

2 tablespoons cacao powder

1 to 2 tablespoons almond butter

1. In a blender, blend the almond milk, avocado, banana, cacao powder, and almond butter.
2. Enjoy this mousse at room temperature right out of the blender, or chill for 20 minutes and serve.

VARIATION TIP: I like to top this mousse with nut butter and hemp hearts or cacao nibs.

PER SERVING Calories: 255; Saturated Fat: 4g; Total Fat: 18g; Protein: 8g; Total Carbs: 30g; Fiber: 12g; Sodium: 175mg

Banana Bread Quinoa Bars

MAKES: 9–12 SERVINGS / PREP TIME: 10 MINUTES / COOK TIME: 25 MINUTES

GLUTEN-FREE, VEGAN

Quinoa is a gluten-free pseudo-grain that is a complete plant-based protein source. Rich in antioxidants and high in fiber, it contains omega-3 fatty acids, which decrease inflammation. Quinoa is incredibly versatile because it takes on the flavor of whatever you cook with it.

½ cup gluten-free rolled oats

½ cup almond flour

½ cup uncooked quinoa, rinsed

1 teaspoon baking powder

1 teaspoon ground cinnamon

Pinch sea salt

2 bananas

½ cup all-natural peanut butter

¼ cup unsweetened applesauce

3 tablespoons ground flaxseed

¼ to ½ cup chocolate chips, for topping (optional)

Chopped nuts, for topping (optional)

Fresh fruit, for topping (optional)

1. Preheat the oven to 350°F. Line an 8-by-8-inch baking dish with parchment paper.
2. In a large bowl, combine the oats, almond flour, quinoa, baking powder, cinnamon, and salt.
3. In a medium bowl, mash the bananas with a fork. Add the peanut butter, applesauce, and flaxseed and stir to combine. Pour the wet mixture into the dry mixture and stir until well combined.
4. Pour the batter into a casserole dish and spread evenly.
5. Bake for 25 minutes, until golden brown on top.
6. Allow the bread to cool for 10 minutes before cutting into bars. Add the desired toppings before serving.

PER SERVING Calories: 151; Saturated Fat: 1g; Total Fat: 8g; Protein: 5g; Total Carbs: 15g; Fiber: 4g; Sodium: 45mg

Chocolate Truffles

MAKES: 12–15 SERVINGS / PREP TIME: 10 MINUTES

GLUTEN-FREE, VEGAN

Almonds are a great source of protein and healthy fats; they contain fiber, which helps control blood sugar levels. Almonds contain magnesium, manganese, calcium, and vitamin E. This fat-soluble vitamin is an antioxidant. If you do not have almonds, you can substitute other nuts or seeds.

¼ cup vegan chocolate protein powder

¼ cup plus
1 tablespoon
cacao powder

⅓ cup unsweetened shredded coconut

¼ cup chopped almonds

2 tablespoons shelled hemp seeds

½ cup plus
2 tablespoons
almond butter

1 tablespoon unsweetened original almond milk

1 teaspoon pure vanilla extract

1. In a large bowl, combine the protein powder, cacao powder, coconut, almonds, hemp seeds, almond butter, almond milk, and vanilla and mix well by hand.
2. Roll into 1-inch balls and serve.

RECIPE TIP: If the mixture seems too dry, add a dash more almond milk and work by hand to mix and roll into balls.

STORAGE TIP: Place in an airtight container and store in the refrigerator for up to five days or freeze for up to one month.

PER SERVING Calories: 177; Saturated Fat: 6g; Total Fat: 15g; Protein: 8g; Total Carbs: 9g; Fiber: 5g; Sodium: 50mg

Chocolate Cookies

MAKES: 20-22 BALLS / **PREP TIME:** 10 MINUTES / **COOK TIME:** 10 MINUTES

GLUTEN-FREE, VEGETARIAN

Make these cookies nut-free by substituting sunflower seed butter for the peanut butter. If you're vegan, use a flaxseed mixture instead of the egg. In a small bowl, mix 3 tablespoons ground flaxseed with ⅓ cup of water. Let the mixture sit for 10 minutes until thickened, then add it to the other ingredients.

⅓ cup cacao powder

¾ teaspoon baking soda

1 cup all-natural peanut butter or any nut or seed butter

1 egg

⅓ cup unsweetened applesauce

1 teaspoon pure vanilla extract

1. Preheat the oven to 350°F. Line a baking sheet with parchment paper.
2. In a large bowl, mix the cacao powder and baking soda. Add the peanut butter, egg, applesauce, and vanilla and mix until just combined. Do not overmix.
3. Scoop the batter into small balls and place on the baking sheet. Flatten slightly with a fork.
4. Bake for 10 to 12 minutes. The cookies should be soft and moist on the inside and crispy on the outside.
5. Let cool for 5 minutes before serving.

STORAGE TIP: Store in an airtight container for up to five days or freeze for up to one month.

VARIATION TIP: You can get creative with add-ins, such as ¼ cup of chopped nuts, seeds, cacao nibs, or coconut flakes.

PER SERVING Calories: 102; Saturated Fat: 2g; Total Fat: 8g; Protein: 4g; Total Carbs: 5g; Fiber: 2g; Sodium: 50mg

Cookie Dough Balls

MAKES: 16–20 BALLS / **PREP TIME:** 10 MINUTES

GLUTEN-FREE, VEGAN

These cookie dough balls are made with chickpeas, which are high in protein and fiber. Chickpeas are a good source of iron, which can be lacking in the diets of vegans and vegetarians.

1 (15.5-ounce) can chickpeas, drained and rinsed

½ cup all-natural almond butter or peanut butter

2 tablespoons Apple Butter (page 86)

¼ cup cacao nibs or chopped nuts (almonds, walnuts, or cashews)

1. In a food processor, blend the chickpeas, almond butter, and apple butter until the mixture resembles cookie dough. Stop periodically to scrape the mixture from the sides.
2. In a large bowl, combine the mixture with the cacao nibs.
3. Roll into 16 to 20 balls. Serve and enjoy.

STORAGE TIP: Store in an airtight container for up to one week or freeze for up to one month.

SUBSTITUTION TIP: If you are off the detox or do not have apple butter available, you can substitute pure honey. You can also replace the cacao nibs with dairy-free chocolate chips.

PER SERVING Calories: 81; Saturated Fat: 1g; Total Fat: 5g; Protein: 3g; Total Carbs: 7g; Fiber: 3g; Sodium: 17mg

Chocolate Seed Bars

MAKES: 15–18 SERVINGS / **PREP TIME:** 10 MINUTES, PLUS
30 MINUTES TO FREEZE / **COOK TIME:** 5 MINUTES

GLUTEN-FREE, VEGAN

Shelled hemp seeds are an excellent source of protein, omega-3 fatty acids, iron, vitamin B_1 (thiamine), phosphorus, magnesium, zinc, and manganese. Be sure to refrigerate them so they won't go rancid.

½ cup coconut oil

½ cup vegan chocolate protein powder

1 teaspoon almond butter

½ cup pumpkin seeds

¼ cup sunflower seeds

¼ cup sesame seeds

¼ cup shelled hemp seeds

1. Line a baking sheet with parchment paper.
2. In a small pot, heat the coconut oil and chocolate protein powder over medium heat. Stir frequently until melted, about 3 minutes. Add the almond butter and mix well.
3. Remove from the heat, add the pumpkin seeds, sunflower seeds, sesame seeds, and hemp seeds, and stir until well combined.
4. Pour the seed mixture onto the baking sheet and spread evenly.
5. Place the sheet in the freezer for about 30 minutes, or until firm. Remove and cut into squares.

STORAGE TIP: Store in an airtight container in the freezer for up to one month.

SUBSTITUTION TIP: If you are missing one of these seeds in your pantry, simply switch for any other seed or nut, such as chopped almonds, pecans, or cashews.

PER SERVING Calories: 132; Saturated Fat: 7g; Total Fat: 12g; Protein: 6g; Total Carbs: 1g; Fiber: 1g; Sodium: 38mg

Chocolate Almond Butter Cups

MAKES: 12 SERVINGS / PREP TIME: 10 MINUTES, PLUS 30 MINUTES
TO FREEZE / COOK TIME: 5 MINUTES

GLUTEN-FREE, VEGAN

Raw cacao is the purest form of chocolate. Rich in fiber, calcium, magnesium, iron, and potassium, cacao is also an excellent source of antioxidants, containing almost 40 times more than blueberries. Studies show that raw cacao releases endorphins that naturally elevate your mood.

½ cup coconut oil

½ cup vegan protein powder

2 teaspoons cacao powder

½ cup natural almond butter or nut butter or ¼ cup chopped almonds

1. Line a muffin tin with liners.
2. In a small pot over medium heat, melt the coconut oil, then stir in the protein powder and cacao powder. Mix well; the powders should dissolve into the coconut oil. Remove from the heat.
3. Pour enough of the cacao mixture to just cover the bottom of each muffin cup (reserving a bit to top), and place 2 teaspoons almond butter in each cup.
4. Top each cup with the remaining cacao mixture.
5. Place in the freezer for 30 minutes, or until solid.

STORAGE TIP: Store in an airtight container for up to three months. Thaw for 5 minutes before eating.

PER SERVING Calories: 166; Saturated Fat: 9g; Total Fat: 15g; Protein: 7g; Total Carbs: 1g; Fiber: 1g; Sodium: 63mg

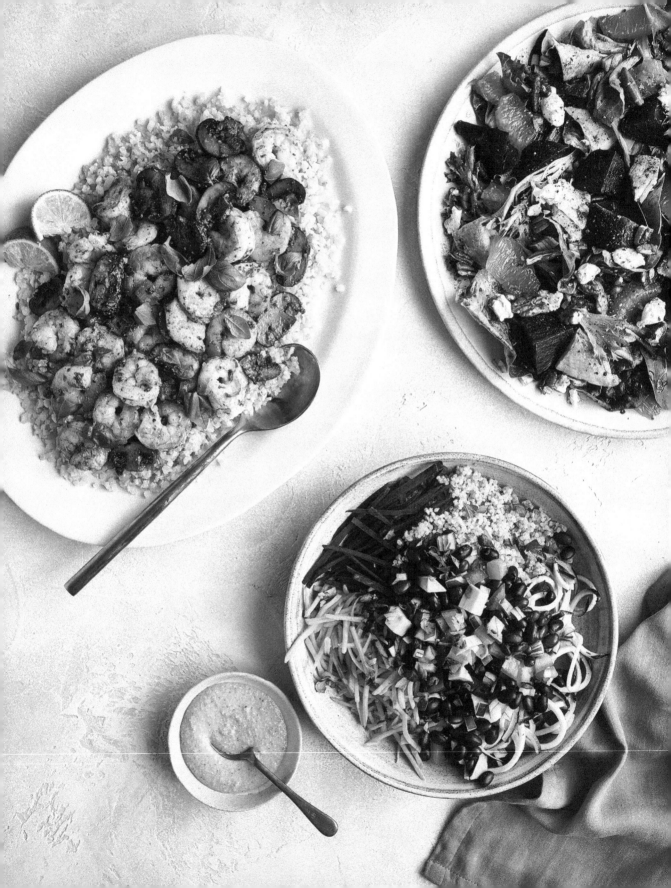

Measurement Conversions

VOLUME EQUIVALENTS (LIQUID)

US STANDARD	US STANDARD (OUNCES)	METRIC (APPROXIMATE)
2 tablespoons	1 fl. oz.	30 mL
¼ cup	2 fl. oz.	60 mL
½ cup	4 fl. oz.	120 mL
1 cup	8 fl. oz.	240 mL
1½ cups	12 fl. oz.	355 mL
2 cups or 1 pint	16 fl. oz.	475 mL
4 cups or 1 quart	32 fl. oz.	1 L
1 gallon	128 fl. oz.	4 L

OVEN TEMPERATURES

FAHRENHEIT (F)	CELSIUS (C) (APPROXIMATE)
250°F	120°C
300°F	150°C
325°F	165°C
350°F	180°C
375°F	190°C
400°F	200°C
425°F	220°C
450°F	230°C

VOLUME EQUIVALENTS (DRY)

US STANDARD	METRIC (APPROXIMATE)
⅛ teaspoon	0.5 mL
¼ teaspoon	1 mL
½ teaspoon	2 mL
¾ teaspoon	4 mL
1 teaspoon	5 mL
1 tablespoon	15 mL
¼ cup	59 mL
⅓ cup	79 mL
½ cup	118 mL
⅔ cup	156 mL
¾ cup	177 mL
1 cup	235 mL
2 cups or 1 pint	475 mL
3 cups	700 mL
4 cups or 1 quart	1 L

WEIGHT EQUIVALENTS

US STANDARD	METRIC (APPROXIMATE)
½ ounce	15 g
1 ounce	30 g
2 ounces	60 g
4 ounces	115 g
8 ounces	225 g
12 ounces	340 g
16 ounces or 1 pound	455 g

References

American Heart Association. "How Much Sugar Is Too Much?" Accessed December 28, 2019. https://www.heart.org/en/healthy-living/healthy-eating /eat-smart/sugar/how-much-sugar-is-too-much.

Brazier, Brendan. *The Thrive Diet, 10th Anniversary Edition: The Plant-based Whole Foods Way to Staying Healthy for Life.* Canada: Penguin, 2017.

Enders, Giulia. *Gut: The Inside Story Of Our Body's Most Underrated Organ.* Vancouver: Greystone Books, 2015.

Frei, B., L. England, and B. N. Ames. "Ascorbate Is an Outstanding Antioxidant in Human Blood Plasma." *Proceedings of the National Academy of Science* 86, no. 16 (1989): 6377–81.

Gottfried, Sara. *Brain Body Diet: 40 Days to a Lean, Calm, Energized, and Happy Self.* New York: HarperCollins, 2019.

Government of Canada. "Fibre." Accessed December 28, 2019. https://www .canada.ca/en/health-canada/services/nutrients/fibre.html.

Horsager, C., S. D. Ostergaard, and M. B. Lauritsen. *The Food Addiction Denmark (FADK) Project.* Cambridge: Cambridge University Press, 2019.

Li, Y., and H. E. Schellhorn. "New Developments and Novel Therapeutic Perspectives for Vitamin C." *Journal of Nutrition* 137 (2007): 2171–84.

McCarthy, Joy. *Joyous Detox: Your Complete Plan and Cookbook To Be Vibrant Daily.* Canada: Penguin House, 2016.

Sanfilippo, Diane. (2018). *The 21 Day Sugar Detox Daily Guide.* Las Vegas: Victory Belt Publishing, 2018.

Schiff, Wendy, and Matthew Durant. *Nutrition for Healthy Living.* Canada: McGraw-Hill Ryerson, 2011.

Index

Acknowledgments

Thank you to you, the reader, and my wonderful online community—I wrote this book for you. Your stories, your online interactions via social media, and meeting you in person all motivated me to write this book to the best of my ability. You inspire me daily to create new, healthy recipes and educational content to help you achieve your health goals. My goal is for you to live your happiest, healthiest life. I want to thank you for supporting my first book and for your continued support, love, encouraging words, and online engagement. I would not be where I am today if it weren't for all of you. I am truly grateful.

Mark: Thank you for being my rock always. It's hard for me to find the words to express just how much I love and respect you. Your unconditional love, help, words of encouragement, and support (I see all the extras you had to do around the house and with the kids to make my dream manifest) are so appreciated. From the bottom of my heart, thank you.

Layla, Sura, and Rowan: I want you to know just how much you inspire me to live my dreams because I want you to live your dreams fearlessly, too. Thank you for all your love, hugs, support, and understanding through the process of writing this book. Most importantly, thank you for always being so open to trying Mommy's new creations and giving me honest feedback on each recipe.

Marcy: Thank you for your continued support of me following my path and continuing to push myself with writing. You are a beautiful guiding light that is always shining bright, and your energy is magnetic.

Corryn, Sam, Shannon, Ashleigh, and Sierra: THANK YOU for being the best everything—friends, cheerleaders, sounding boards, and support systems throughout this process. I look up to all of you and appreciate your feedback, encouragement, hugs, ideas, and inspiration.

Tanya: thank you for your help and support for this book. You are a great foodie friend and I just wanted to let you know that I appreciate you.

Amanda, Sarah, and Tanya: You ladies are forever my soul sisters. Thank you for always being there to support my vision and dreams unconditionally.

Daniel: Thank you for all of your advice and edits for this book; I appreciate all of your guidance and assistance.

About the Author

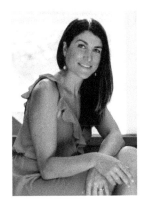

Pam Rocca is a vibrant nutritionist and health coach who is passionate about simplifying health and healthy eating and making it accessible for everyone. Her infectious energy has been creating a movement toward adding more fun and joy in the kitchen and making food that not only tastes delicious, but looks and smells awesome, too. She loves to create and share new nutritious recipes that are easy to follow on both her blog and in her cookbooks. With three spunky children she knows firsthand how hard it can be to get a good meal on the table that the whole family can enjoy. From her own struggles with food, health, and nutrition and a whole lot of trial and error, she has come up with a way of eating that nourishes your body from the inside out. Pam is fiercely committed to supporting others to fuel their bodies in a way that allows them to live their best life. Pam works with women as a health coach to promote healthy relationships with food and body image from a place of self-love. Pam lives in Barrie, Ontario, with her husband, Mark; their daughters, Layla and Sura; and son, Rowan. Her blog can be found online at pamrocca.com. Follow her journey on Instagram to see what she's creating each week at @pam_rocca.

CPSIA information can be obtained
at www.ICGtesting.com
Printed in the USA
JSHW061409080922
30227JS00003B/6